Public Health in the 21st Century

Anal Fissure

Symptoms, Diagnosis and Treatment

PUBLIC HEALTH IN THE 21ST CENTURY

Additional books in this series can be found on Nova's website under the Series tab.

Additional E-books in this series can be found on Nova's website under the E-books tab.

PUBLIC HEALTH IN THE 21ST CENTURY

ANAL FISSURE

SYMPTOMS, DIAGNOSIS AND TREATMENT

PIERPAOLO SILERI
AND
ACHILLE LUCIO GASPARI
EDITORS

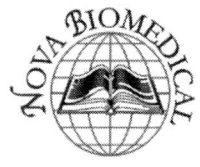

Nova Science Publishers, Inc.
New York

Copyright © 2012 by Nova Science Publishers, Inc.

All rights reserved. No part of this book may be reproduced, stored in a retrieval system or transmitted in any form or by any means: electronic, electrostatic, magnetic, tape, mechanical photocopying, recording or otherwise without the written permission of the Publisher.

For permission to use material from this book please contact us:
Telephone 631-231-7269; Fax 631-231-8175
Web Site: http://www.novapublishers.com

NOTICE TO THE READER

The Publisher has taken reasonable care in the preparation of this book, but makes no expressed or implied warranty of any kind and assumes no responsibility for any errors or omissions. No liability is assumed for incidental or consequential damages in connection with or arising out of information contained in this book. The Publisher shall not be liable for any special, consequential, or exemplary damages resulting, in whole or in part, from the readers' use of, or reliance upon, this material. Any parts of this book based on government reports are so indicated and copyright is claimed for those parts to the extent applicable to compilations of such works.

Independent verification should be sought for any data, advice or recommendations contained in this book. In addition, no responsibility is assumed by the publisher for any injury and/or damage to persons or property arising from any methods, products, instructions, ideas or otherwise contained in this publication.

This publication is designed to provide accurate and authoritative information with regard to the subject matter covered herein. It is sold with the clear understanding that the Publisher is not engaged in rendering legal or any other professional services. If legal or any other expert assistance is required, the services of a competent person should be sought. FROM A DECLARATION OF PARTICIPANTS JOINTLY ADOPTED BY A COMMITTEE OF THE AMERICAN BAR ASSOCIATION AND A COMMITTEE OF PUBLISHERS.

Additional color graphics may be available in the e-book version of this book.

Library of Congress Cataloging-in-Publication Data

Anal fissure : symptoms, diagnosis and treatment / editors, Pierpaolo Sileri and Achille Lucio Gaspari.
   p. ; cm.
 Includes bibliographical references and index.
 ISBN 978-1-61209-716-9 (softcover : alk. paper)
 1. Anus--Diseases. 2. Anus--Diseases--Treatment. I. Sileri, Pierpaolo. II. Gaspari, Achille.
 [DNLM: 1. Fissure in Ano--therapy. 2. Fissure in Ano--diagnosis. WI 605]
 RC866.A53 2011
 616.3'5--dc22
                              2011009052

Published by Nova Science Publishers, Inc. † New York

Contents

Preface		vii
List of Contributors		ix
Chapter 1	Anal Canal: Anatomy and Phisiopathology *Michele Grande*	1
Chapter 2	Chemical Sphincterotomy *Giovanni Milito and Federica Cadeddu*	29
Chapter 3	Botulinum Toxin and Anal Fissure *Oliver Jones*	47
Chapter 4	Current Surgical Management of Anal Fissure *Jason W. Allen and Herand Abcarian*	63
Chapter 5	Postoperative Complications after Treatment for Chronic Anal Fissure *Giovanni Milito, Federica Cadeddu and Ilaria Ciangola*	75
Chapter 6	Anal Fissure: Treatment Options in Particular Cases *Stefano D'Ugo, Sara Di Carlo, Lodovico Patrizi and Vito Maria Stolfi*	91

Chapter 7	Conservative and Surgical Treatment of Chronic Anal Fissure: Longer-Term Results from our Prospective Database *Pierpaolo Sileri, Luana Franceschilli, Giulio P. Angelucci, Sara Lazzaro, Alessandra Di Giorgio, and Achille L. Gaspari*	**105**
Index		**123**

PREFACE

Anal fissure is a common problem with a prevalence in the general population around 2%.

However this rate is underestimated, being probably as high as 15%, since most symptomatic patients do not seek medical attention and prefer self-treatments usually erroneous secondary to misdiagnosis.

The presence of an anal fissure is reliably associated with an elevated intra-anal pressure and decreased blood flow to the anoderm. Symptoms include pain, bleeding, pruritus, and soiling. Greater than 90% of acute anal fissures are of short duration and heal spontaneously or with simple measures. A high-fiber diet with an increased intake of water is recommended, laxatives may be used when required to make soft constipated stool and warm sitz baths may offer symptomatic relief. Acute fissures that fail to heal become chronic fissures, which have traditionally been treated by surgery.

Traditionally, lateral internal sphincterotomy has been considered the gold standard treatment for chronic fissures, but this procedure requires anaesthesia and is associated with a noteworthy risk of incontinence. More recently, various pharmacologic agents have been shown to decrease resting anal pressure and promote fissure healing. This so-called *chemical sphincterotomy* has been used as first-line treatment for chronic anal fissure in many centres.

The authors of this book review and discuss recent developments on anal fissure conservative medical and surgical treatment as well as the management of surgical complications. This books, through the personal experience of all contributors, offers a complete guide to general practitioner, resident and medical student who frequently face with difficult questions concerning the optimum management of anal fissure.

LIST OF CONTRIBUTORS

Herand Abcarian
Professor of Surgery
University of Illinois at Chicago, Chicago, IL, US

Jason W. Allen
Clinical Fellow, Surgery
University of Illinois at Chicago, Chicago, IL, US

Giulio Paolo Angelucci
Research Yellow, Surgery
University of Rome Tor Vergata, Rome, Italy

Ilaria Ciangola
Resident in General Surgery
University of Rome Tor Vergata, Rome, Italy

Federica Cadeddu
Assistant Professor of Surgery
University of Rome Tor Vergata, Rome, Italy

Stefano D'Ugo
Resident in General Surgery
University of Rome Tor Vergata, Rome, Italy

Sara Di Carlo
Resident in General Surgery
University of Rome Tor Vergata, Rome, Italy

Luana Franceschilli
Clinical Fellow, Colorectal Surgery
University of Rome Tor Vergata, Rome, Italy

Michele Grande
Assistant Professor Surgery
University of Rome Tor Vergata, Rome, Italy

Oliver Jones
Consultant Surgeon
John Radcliffe Hospital, Oxford, United Kingdom

Sara Lazzaro
Research Fellow, Surgery
University of Rome Tor Vergata, Rome, Italy

Giovanni Milito
Associate Professor of Surgery
University of Rome Tor Vergata, Rome, Italy

Lodovico Patrizi
Assistant Professor of Gynecology and Obstetrics
University of Rome Tor Vergata, Rome, Italy

Vito Maria Stolfi
Associate Professor Surgery
University of Rome Tor Vergata, Rome, Italy

In: Anal Fissure
Editors: P. Sileri and A. L. Gaspari

ISBN: 978-1-61209-716-9
© 2012 Nova Science Publishers, Inc

Chapter 1

ANAL CANAL: ANATOMY AND PHYSIOPATHOLOGY

Michele Grande
University of Rome Tor Vergata, Rome, Italy

ANATOMY

The Anal Canal

The term "anal canal" was proposed by Symington in 1888 to indicate the portion "perineal" rectum, limited by the pelvic floor up and anal orifice down [1]. This definition corresponds to that given by Morgan and Thompson (1956) of surgical anal canal, extended from anorectal ring to the anal margin, which differs from the anatomical anal canal, between the dentate line and anal margin [2].

The dentate line, located at the midpoint or middle third of the union with the lower third of the internal sphincter, it refers to the line of anal valves [3]. These valves, semilunar in appearance, sometimes papillary, connect the base columns of Morgagni, arranged into 6-10 vertical folds, with circumferential distribution around the lumen of the anal canal [4], which are particularly evident to just below the midpoint of the anal canal, gradually disappearing at the upper end of that. Opening into these crypts are a variable number of anal glands that traverse the submucosa to enter the internal sphincter and terminate in the intersphincteric plane, exocrine structures that cross the internal sphincter, in some cases reach the intersphinteric plane, and help to lubricate the anal canal [5]. Among the many synonyms used to indicate the line of anal valves (pectinate line, the line of crypts, papillary line, line ano-cutaneous, muco-cutaneous junction, anorectal line) the term of the dentate line seems to be the most correct, its approximate distance from the anal margin is about 2 cm [6,7, 8,9,10,11]. The term "anorectal ring" was introduced by Milligan and Morgan (1934) to indicate to this muscular ring at the junction of the rectum with the anal canal, very important from a functional point of view; consist of internal sphincter completed by muscle puborectal for the upper half and the external sphincter for the lower half. Between internal and external sphincter is inter-sphincteric space with the longitudinal layer (Figure 1) [3,12].

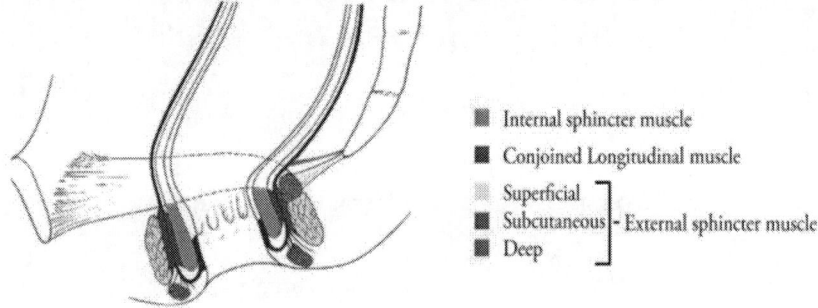

Figure 1. Schematic representation of the anal sphincter.

The anal margin is defined as the point at which the walls of the anal canal come into contact in their normal resting position. If the histological anal canal extends from top to the bottom of internal sphincter inside a length of about 3 cm, in living anorectal ring distance from the anal margin (anal orifice) is about 4 cm [7,13,14]. It is therefore appropriate, taking into account the influence of fixation procedures on real measures of histological samples, to match approximately the anal margin to intersphincteric groove, between the edge of the internal sphincter muscle and the distal portion (subcutaneous) of the external sphincter, near which there is the passage from epithelium of the anal canal to the perianal skin [10].

Although the term of ano-cutaneous line, synonymous board or anal margin, may, according to some authors, give rise to confusion in clinical practice is widely used [15,8,10]. The anal orifice in males is behind the line of ischial spine, at 20-25 mm from apex of the coccyx, while in woman is more superficial and coincides with line of ischial spine, at 25-30 mm from apex of the coccyx [16].

Histologically, the anal canal has a variable lining. The mucosa of the upper anal canal, like that of the rectum, is lined by columnar epithelium. There is a transitional or cloacogenic zone where the mucosa consists of layers of cuboid cells interspersed with tongues of columnar epithelium. The mucosa distal to the dentate line is lined by squamous epithelium devoid of hair and glands [17]. At the anal verge, the lining acquires the characters of normal skin with its apocrine glands.

The area with transitional epithelium has been shown over time with different names (mucosal zone, middle zone, cloacal region, hemorrhoidal zone, transitional zone), the term "anal transitional zone" (ATZ), recently introduced, seems to be better corresponding to its characteristics: this is indeed an area interposed between a colorectal mucosa proximal and squamous epithelium distally.

Its extension is variable: from a few millimeters to 2 cm above (usually 1 cm) and a few millimeters to ½ cm below the dentate line. In ATZ may contain areas of squamous epithelium, simple columnar or colorectal cryptic, melanocytes and endocrine cells, Paneth cells, islands of pyloric metaplasia and gastric mucosa of fundic type; frequently the epithelium of ATZ consists of cells can be columnar, cuboidal, polygonal and flat arranged in 4-9 layers [8].

The anal canal, surrounded by levator ani and sphincters, is connected posteriorly to the apex of the coccyx and the raphe or ligament anococcigeo. This ligament, tense between the rear of the anal canal and the coccyx, is formed from the crossing of fibers from both sides of the elevator and below the confluence of the external sphincter fibers that are attached to the coccyx [18].

Lateral to the external sphincter lies the ischioanal space. The triangular ischioanal space is bordered superiorly by the levator ani muscle. Posteriorly, the most caudal space is the superficial postanal space that terminates at the coccyx. Above the superficial postanal space is the anococcygeal ligament, and deep to this ligament, but below the levator ani muscle is the deep postanal space (space of Courtney) (Figure 2). This space is continuous laterally with each ischioanal space and when infected can create a large ''horseshoe'' abscess. Above the levator ani, below and posterior to the rectum, and anterior and superior to the sacrum is the supralevator space that can extend into the retroperitoneum (17). Before the anal canal in males is related with the tendinous center of perineum, the urogenital diaphragm that contains the membranous portion of the urethra and the bulbous urethra; in women with perineal body and posterior vaginal wall.

The mucosa of the anal canal that extends above the dentate line adheres loosely to the underlying muscle (internal sphincter) interposing between the two structures submucosal space containing the internal hemorrhoidal plexus, which continues proximally with the submucosa of the rectum. This space is limited below by the suspensory ligament of Parks, located at the halfway down the anal canal, composed of fibers that, coming from the internal sphincter and the muscularis mucosae is set at the level of the crypts, the lining of the anal canal causing a strong anchored to the surface muscle [19].

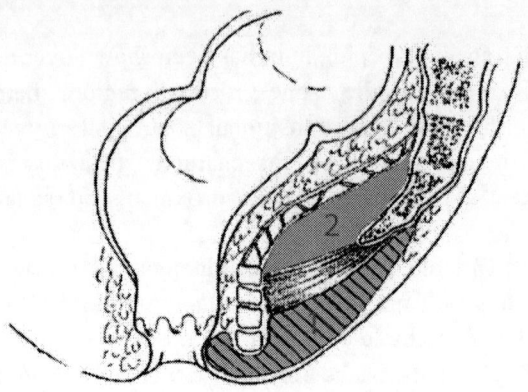

Figure 2. Postanal space: sagittal section. 1, superficial postanal space; 2, deep postanal space (space of Courtney).

Anal sphincter continence involving three muscles: internal sphincter (involuntary), external sphincter (voluntary) and levator ani.

A recent study of 20 normal subjects showed, by using three-dimensional endoanal ultrasonography, that there are differences between the sexes regarding the anatomy sphincter [20]. The anal canal was longer in males (32.6 ± 5.3 mm) than in women (25.1 ± 3.4mm, P = 0.001). Similarly, in the male internal anal sphincter was found to be longer (25.6 ± 6.3 mm) than in women (19.8 ± 4.0 mm, P = 0.02), even if the length of the internal sphincter as percentage of the total length of the anal channel did not show differences in both sexes (78.3 ± 8.2% and 78.7 ± 9.0% in male and female, respectively, P = 0.91).

The internal sphincter is not merely a thickened extension of the circular smooth muscle layer surrounding the colon. Indeed, in dogs, the rectal circular muscle layer is tightly packed with poorly defined septa while the internal anal sphincter contains discrete muscle bundles separated by large septa [21]. In the rectum, the interstitial cells of Cajal (ICC) are organized in dense networks along the submucosal and myenteric borders. In the internal anal sphincter, the ICCs are located along the periphery of the muscle bundles within the circular layer [21].

The internal sphincter extend up to a length of about 3 cm and have a thickness between 2 and 8 mm [22]; its lower limit is about 6-8 mm anal orifice [3,23]. It is innervated by fibers of the autonomic nervous system and delivering with its involuntary contraction continence.

The inter-sphincteric space is a thin fat-containing space with variable thickness: it may be hard to discern in some and easily visible in others. The inter-sphincteric space contains the longitudinal layer (also named longitudinal muscle), which is the continuation of the smooth muscle longitudinal layer of the rectum. The longitudinal layer receives contributions from the levator ani, particularly the puboanalis, and a large fibro-elastic element derived from the endopelvic fascia. The longitudinal layer is 2.5 mm thick and the thickness decreases with age. Cranially the layer is predominantly muscular while fibro-elastic caudally. The fibro-elastic tissue of the longitudinal layer is continuous with the fibro-elastic network outside the sphincter to the perianal skin to form the corrugator cutis ani, thereby forming an intra-sphincteric fibro-elastic network passing through the external sphincter [24].

Shafik supports a different morphological organization of the anal longitudinal muscle. The author believes that this muscle is composed of three layers separated by fascial septa: the medial layer is an extension of the longitudinal muscle of the rectum, the intermediate is an extension of the elevator ani (pubococcygeus muscle) while the lateral, present only in the lower part of the anal canal, is an extension of the deep portion of the external sphincter. At the lower internal sphincter these three layers form a common central tendon from which branch off some fibers crossing the distal portion (subcutaneous) of the external sphincter and, below it, are attached on the perianal skin to form the corrugator cutis ani [3,8,25].

The external sphincter consists of striated muscle fibres, and according to recent studies also a component of smooth muscle, surrounding an elliptical or circular course the anal canal, lateral to the internal sphincter muscle and the muscle longitudinal [26]. The external sphincter is approximately 2.7 cm high, but is anteriorly shorter in women (approximately 1.5 cm) [3]. The lateral part of the external sphincter is approximately 2.7 cm high. The external sphincter has a thickness of 4 mm on endoluminal imaging [24] . MRI studies have made clear that the external sphincter forms the lower outer part of the anal sphincter and the puborectalis the upper outer part [24].

Number of its components, two (superficial and deep) [27,28,29,30] or three (one subcutaneous, superficial and deep) is still discussed [12,15].

An interesting theory of functional organization of the external sphincter in three slings muscle action opposed was proposed by Shafik. The external sphincter is considered to have three muscle groups willing to sling around the anal canal, these slings, proceeding in the craniocaudal may display a convexity respectively front, rear and then front again. The upper muscle group would be composed by the deep layer of the sphincter and bundles puborectal, attached below to the pubis. The intermediate group was constituted by the surface layer of the sphincter, anchored to the dorsal surface of the apex of the coccyx. The third identified with the sling portion subcutaneously, anchored before the perianal skin and crossed by longitudinal muscle fibres (Figure 3) [31].

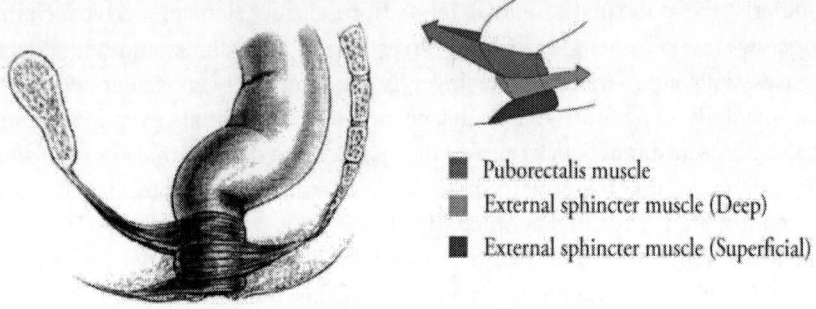

Figure 3. Schematic representation of triple tie of Shafik.

Theories Shafik, very interesting, have been subject to criticism, and have not been confirmed in subsequent studies [3,7,32,33]. Currently it is considered that the external sphincter has posterior fibres continuous with the anococcygeal ligament, some of the anterior fibres decussate into the superficial transverse perineal muscles and perineal body. The deep part of the external sphincter is intimately related to the puborectalis [24].

Lateral to the external sphincter lays the ischioanal space. The triangular ischioanal space is bordered superiorly by the levator ani muscle. Posteriorly, the most caudal space is the superficial postanal space that terminates at the coccyx. Above the superficial postanal space is the anococcygeal ligament, and deep to this ligament, but below the levator ani muscle is the deep postanal space (space of Courtney). This space is continuous laterally with each ischioanal space and when infected can create a large "horseshoe" abscess. Above the levator ani, below and posterior to the rectum, and anterior and superior to the sacrum is the supralevator space that can extend into the retroperitoneum [17].

Pelvic Floor Muscles

The levator ani separates the pelvic cavity from the perineum and performs the dual function of supporting the visceral organs and maintaining continence. It originates from the posterior surface of the superior pubic rami bilaterally and attaches to the inner surface of the ischium. Traditionally the levator ani muscle has been thought to consist of 3 muscles: (1) the iliococcygeal muscle, (2) the pubococcygeal muscle, and (3) the puborectalis muscle.

- The iliococcygeus arises from the posterior half of the tendineus arc inserting into the last two segments of the coccyx and the midline anococcygeal raphe. The anococcygeal raphe is the interdigitation of the iliococcygeal fibres from both sides and extends from the coccyx to the anorectal junction. The iliococcygeus forms a sheet-like layer and is often largely aponeurotic. Carries a support on the back of the anal canal, without contracting a direct relationship with the rectal wall;
- The pubococcygeus arises from the anterior half of the tendineus arc and the periosteum of the posterior surface of the pubic bone at the lower border of the pubic symphysis, its fibres directed posteriorly inserting into the anococcygeal raphe and coccyx;
- The puborectalis forms a U-shaped sling around the urogenital hiatus. Contraction of the puborectalis lifts and compresses the urogenital hiatus. The puborectalis is the main part of this muscle and goes around the upper part of the anus where it is attached posteriorly to the anococcygeal ligament. During vaginal delivery the levator ani muscle is substantially stretched and injury may occur, often near the pubic bone insertion [27,29].

According to recent interpretations levator ani is formed by iliococcygeus and pubococcygeus, while puborectal be considered as part of the deep portion of the external sphincter, both are supplied by the pudendal nerve [34,35]; on the contrary electrophysiological studies indicate a direct innervation by branches sacral (S3 and S4), and recent anatomical studies (which in this innervation from the pelvic side include fibers from S2), argue against the thesis of the puborectal innervation by the pudendal nerve [36,37,38].

To mention the coccygeus muscle that forms the posterior part of the pelvic diaphragm. This shelf-like triangular musculotendinous structure has its origin at the ischial spine and courses along the posterior margin of the internal obturator muscle. The muscles inserts at the lateral side of the coccyx and the lowest part of the sacrum. The sacrospinous ligament is at the posterior edge of the coccygeus muscle and is fused with this muscle. The proportions of the muscular and ligamentous parts may vary. The coccygeus is not part of the levator ani, having a different function and origin. The coccygeus muscle is innervated by the third and fourth sacral spinal nerves on its superior surface (24).

Unlike other striated muscles the elevator ani has resting electric activity. Recent studies have suggested that this activity might be a function of intra-abdominal pressure and visceral weight. The activity increase in the erect compared to the recumbent position, and upon elevation of intra-abdominal pressure [39]. The cause of this myoelectric activity is not precisely known, but has been suggested to be related to the presence (in the cadavers) of smooth muscle bundles in the elevator ani [39]. Smooth muscle bundles begin to appear at the lateral part of the elevator ani and gradually increase medially, so that the medial part of the muscle is formed of two layers: deep (pelvic), consisting of smooth muscle bundles, and superficial (perineal) consisting of skeletal fibers. The connective tissue separating the layers serves not only to bind the muscle layers, but seems also to provide a pathway for a neurovascular bundle that supplies the elevator ani muscle.

Arterial Supply

The vascularization of the rectum and anal canal depends by superior, middle and lower rectal (hemorrhoidal) arteries with the contribution of small branches of the middle sacral artery and transverse perineal artery [40]. The inferior mesenteric artery, to the junction with the left common iliac vessels, according to some authors [3, 7,15] or distal to the last sigmoid artery according to other changes the name in superior rectal artery [6,16]. The final branch of the aorta before its bifurcation, descending into the mesorectum with the presacral nerve, terminates inferiorly in the upper portion of the posterior wall of the rectum at the level of the third sacral vertebra where it divides into two branches, right and left. This supplies the rectum and the upper third of the anal canal (Figure 4) [17].

It's possible that by the superior rectal artery origins third median branch called dorsal hemorrhoidal artery or azygous rectum [16]. In some cases the superior rectal artery can be replaced by more arterial branches that arise directly from inferior mesenteric artery distal sigmoid artery [16].

The superior rectal artery main branches divide further into smaller branches that penetrate in the submucosa about 8 cm from the anal margin, and shall run vertically, reach the columns of Morgagni, ending in a capillary plexus at level of the anal valves [41,42]. Some small terminal branches form anastomoses with the submucosal hemorrhoidal plexus other small branches attributable to the superior rectal artery be opened without the interposition of capillaries in the vascular space called the corpus cavernosum of the rectum [43].

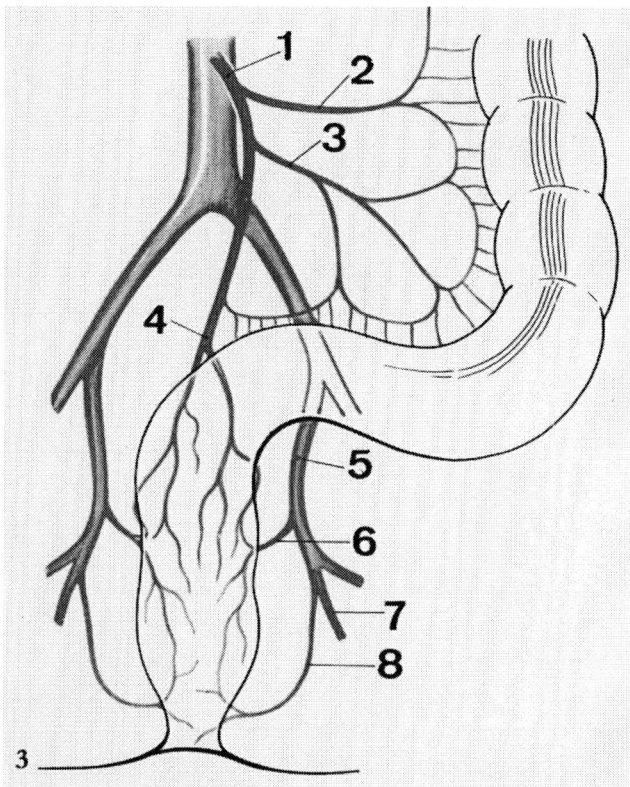

Figure 4. Schematic representation of the vascularization of the rectum and anus. 1, inferior mesenteric artery; 2, left colic artery; 3, sigmoid arteries; 4, superior hemorrhoidal artery; 5, hypogastric artery; 6, middle hemorrhoidal artery; 7, internal pudendal artery; 8, inferior hemorrhoidal artery.

The middle rectal (hemorrhoidal) arteries, originating from the internal iliac arteries, supply to distal rectum and proximal anal canal. The presence of these arteries is variable. The inferior rectal (hemorrhoidal) arteries arise from the internal pudendal artery, which is a branch of the internal iliac artery. These arteries traverse the ischioanal fossa on both sides of the anal canal feeding the sphincter muscles. Intramural collaterals exist between the superior and inferior rectal arteries at the level of the dentate line in the submucosa. This accounts for the low incidence of rectal ischemia [42].

According to a recent study intramural anastomoses exist only between superior and lower rectal artery in the submucosa at the level of dentate line [44].

Unlike the small intestine and colon, which showing on the wall antimesenteric a reduced vascularization and an organization in intramural arterial arches, the arterial network of the rectum is homogeneous and the terminal branches being straight is running for the most part obliquely [42].

Venous Drainage

The veins that drain the rectum and anal canal have a course similar to that of the corresponding arteries. The superior rectal veins tributaries of the portal system via the inferior mesenteric vein, draining the rectum and upper anal canal. The lowermost portion of the rectum and the anal canal drain into the internal iliac veins directly through the middle rectal veins and the inferior rectal veins (via the pudendal vein) [17].

Lymphatic Drainage

Much of the lymphatic drainage of the anal canal and rectum follows the arterial supply. The rectum drains via the superior rectal lymphatics to the inferior mesenteric lymph nodes in the retroperitoneum and laterally to the internal iliac nodes along the middle and inferior rectal vessels through the ischioanal fossa. Lymph drainage from below the dentate line drains to the inguinal nodes. The study of lymphatic drainage in normal anatomy of the rectum revealed the rectal drainage via the superior rectal and inferior mesenteric vessels to the lumboaortic nodes that have no communication with to the internal iliac nodes. However, if distal obstruction occurs, drainage can occur from the anal canal to the superior rectal nodes or laterally to the ischioanal fossa [17].

Innervation

The anorectum and pelvic floor are supplied by sympathetic, parasympathetic and somatic fibres [21].
Sympathetic preganglionic fibres originate from the first 3 lumbar segments of the spinal cord are responsible for innervation of the rectum. After leaving the lumbar region, they join at the preaortic plexus and extend caudally from the aortic bifurcation toward the mesenteric plexus before reaching the level of the upper rectum. It then bifurcates into the left and right branches, traveling down both sides of the pelvis before joining the parasympathetic nerve branches. The parasympathetic nerve supply originates from the caudal 3 sacral nerve roots,

which form the nervi erigentes. The fibers then rapidly progress anteriorly, joining the sympathetic fibers to create the pelvic plexus. The pelvic plexus is located laterally and superior to the levator ani muscle in the mid portion of the lateral stalk. The pelvic plexus then feeds the urinary and genital organs and the rectum with both parasympathetic and sympathetic fibers (Figure 5) [21].

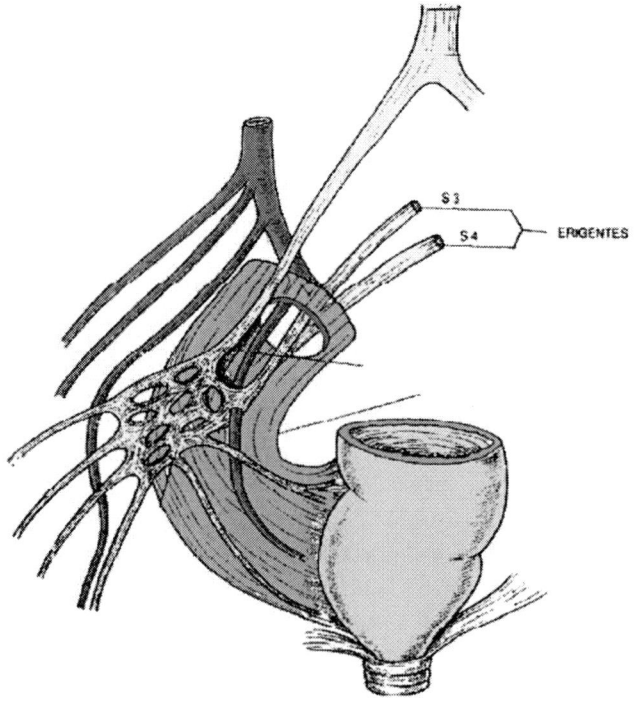

Figure 5. Schematic representation of the pelvic plexus.

The pelvic plexus also supplies the periprostatic plexus that is important for sexual function in men [45].

In women, the hypogastric plexus composed of sympathetic nerve fibers pass through the uterosacral ligament near the rectum. In men, these fibers pass adjacent to the anterolateral wall of the rectum in the retroperitoneal tissue. The pudendal nerves arise from the caudal 3 sacral nerve roots. The nerves cross the ischial tuberosity in the lateral wall of the ischioanal fossa bilaterally. It branches into the inferior rectal, perineal, and dorsal nerves of the penis or clitoris [17,45].

The anal canal also receives innervation from both sympathetic and parasympathetic fibers. Both inhibit the internal anal sphincter. The external sphincter relies on innervation from the perineal branch of the fourth sacral nerve and the inferior rectal branch of the internal pudendal nerve. As previously mentioned, the levator ani muscle is innervated by branches of the pudendal, inferior rectal, perineal, and sacral (S3 and S4) nerves [46]. Sensation of the anal canal comes from the inferior rectal nerve, also a branch of the pudendal nerve. The epithelium of the anal canal is extensively innervated up to 2 cm proximal to the dentate line [17].

The myenteric plexus (Auerbach) along with the submucosal (Meissner) form innervation "intrinsic" or enteric plexus. This consists of groups of nerve cells that are located between the circular and the longitudinal muscle layer (Auerbach's plexus) and in the submucosa (Meissner's plexus) from esophagus to the rectum and the anal canal, until the transition zone, below it disappears completely. In the enteric plexus terminating fibers "extrinsic" sympathetic and parasympathetic [23,41]

ANAL SPHINCTER TONE AND REFLEXES

The study of the function of anal sphincters and pelvic floor has been a major boost in recent years, partly due to increased interest in anorectal disease and partly to developments in surgical techniques, which today can significantly reduce the possibility of a colostomy definitive [47].

Fecal continence and defecation are dependent on several neurological and anatomical factors that involve coordinated physiological processes, including intestinal transit and absorbition, colic transit, rectal compliance, expulsion force and coordinated pelvic floor function [48]. Moreover anal continence relies upon the ability of the anorectum to discriminate between the states of fecal matter, solid, liquid, or gas. Its presence also depends on both voluntary and involuntary control and a multitude of other factors, adding to its complexity [17].

The function of reservoir is instead attributable to the adaptability of the rectum with faecal increasing volumes without endorectal pressure increases proportionally. This is possible thanks to the considerable distensibility of the rectum, the result of its structure and properties of highly flexible arrangement of the component muscle relaxing two new volumes. In fact, after initial and rapid increase in intraluminal pressure, probably due to a reflex contraction of the rectal muscles, we see a sharp decrease in pressure which becomes constant in relation to the coefficient of elasticity parietal [49]. Depending on the degree of rectal distension sensitivity changes from its initial filling sensation (sensation first) becomes a constant feeling that lasts about 30 seconds (constant sensation), since to achieve a feeling of urgent need to defecate (maximum tolerable volume). The measurement of volumes and pressures endorectal, measured at those feelings, offers an index of rectal distensibility calculated by Arhan and colleagues by measuring the relationship between stool volume and pressure (compliance) [50].

The smooth muscle internal anal sphincter is formed by a thickening of the circular muscle layer of the rectum [47,51]. The internal muscle layer of the rectum, the circular, which is in direct continuation with the circular muscle of the sigmoid, distally, specializes in the formation of internal anal sphincter, at the pectinate line for a distance of about 2-3 cm occupies a thickness of 0.5-1 cm.

Longitudinal muscle layer, however, is to operate and to break down the fibers of the internal and external sphincters, the so-called longitudinal muscle intersphincteric.

The muscle is innervated by sympathetic and parasympathetic fibers from the intramural non-adrenergic, cholinergic, but neither type purinergic or peptidergic. The sympathetic innervation is through hypogastric nerves and originates from the fifth lumbar segment. This innervation is considered important in maintaining basal tone pressure; denervation reduces, but does not abolish, the contractile activity of the internal anal sphincter, which is therefore also reflect intrinsic myogenic activity. The parasympathetic innervation is supplied by fibers passing through the S2-S4 sacral plexus to the pelvic plexus before and then seem to have little importance in the basal tone while inducing a mild relaxation of internal anal sphincter [52,53]

Duthie and Watts first showed that the intra-anal pressure at rest (by measuring the pressure before and after administration of a releasing muscle) is primarily due to the action of the anal sphincter internal 10. The other contributors to anal resting tone include the external anal sphincter, the anal mucosal folds and the puborectalis muscle. Penninckx et al. estimated that anal resting tone was generated by nerve-induced activity in the internal sphincter (45% of anal resting tone), myogenic tone in the internal sphincter (10%), the external sphincter (35%) and the anal hemorrhoidal plexus (15%) [55]. These figures should be regarded as estimates, because they were obtained, in part, from complex studies, moreover the relative contributions of these factors to anal resting tone are influenced by several factors [21]. This activity sphincter basal or basal tone, it creates a high pressure zone that extends about 4 cm from the ano-cutaneous line up to about 1-1.5 cm above the pectinate line and the peak pressure which is recorded at about 2.5 cm from the line itself. The adjustable pressure within the anal canal, while showing large individual variations (25 to 80 cm H2O), is still significantly higher than those prevailing in the rectum during the resting phase (2-5 cm H2O), this difference is called the anorectal pressure gradient [56,57,58].

Postural changes and other increases in intra-abdominal pressure such as sneezing, coughing, and the Valsava maneuver increase the resting tone of the external sphincter by an anal reflex. The second sacral spinal segment modulates the external sphincter, which can be contracted voluntarily for 40 to 60 second periods [17]. Lower the contribution of the external anal sphincter tone at baseline: in fact, blockade of bilateral pudendal nerves that innervate the external anal sphincter results in a reduction of only 16-20% of muscle tone at rest [59].

Anal resting pressure is not stationary but varies during the day. In addition to spontaneous relaxation of the internal sphincter, circadian variations that are dependent on the sleep-wake cycle and ultradian (~20-40 min in length) rhythms that are independent of the sleep-awake cycle have also been described [21]. These rhythmic oscillations are distinct in contractions of prolonged duration with average frequency of 12.2/min and ultraslow with average frequency of 2.6/min.

Anal relaxation induced by rectal distention (recto-anal inhibitory reflex, RAIR) is mediated by intrinsic nerves, physiologically arrival of the fecal mass in the rectum results in a reduction of the pressure existing in the upper portion of the anal canal. As a consequence of the latter, the waste moves further down and comes into contact with receptors in the upper part of the anal canal. The receptors determine the quality of the content (the sampling reflex). If the time is right for defecation, impulses are sent to further contract the rectal muscles, relax the external sphincter and the pelvic floor with the puborectalis sling, to facilitate defecation.

If defecation has to be suppressed, a voluntary contraction of the external sphincter and pelvic floor, using the puborectalis sling, propels the luminal contents back up again above the rectum and the urge to defecate ceases.

The mechanism of accommodation is guided by spinal reflexes controlled by the cerebral cortex. The first stimulus to defecation occurs in the presence of a volume of approximately 25% of the maximum tolerable, from a filling of 150 ml, the internal sphincter does not take its tone and thus remains in a state of relaxation. Approximately for 350 ml also the tonic activity of the external sphincter is inhibited and continence can be maintained even for a short time with the activity of phasic voluntary contraction.

Under normal conditions, therefore, the internal anal sphincter is in a state of partial contraction and release the response to rectal distension (recto-sphincteric reflex). This tonic contraction partially regulated by a prevailing myogenic component, is supported and modulates by sympathetic, that from V lumbar segment reaches the sphincter through the hypogastric nerves. In histological preparations of the smooth sphincter contraction is mediated by α-adrenergic receptors and released from β [60].

The first population of receptors is predominant, so that the contractile response to noradrenaline can be converted into relaxation when selectively block α-receptors. Acetylcholine, in contrast, by the action on muscarinic receptors shows a predominantly inhibitory effect.

External anal sphincter and pelvic floor muscles show electrical activity at rest (action potentials recordable EMG), this capacity is maintained at subconscious during sleep and varies during position changes. This electrical activity is greater in the upright posture [21].

The anatomical substrate of this function is given by the two types of muscle fibres constituting the striated sphincter apparatus, type 1 fibers suitable for tonic contractions (fatigue resistant, slow twitch) and type 2 fibers suitable for rapid contractions. The fibers distribution favours tonic activity; type 1 predominate in the human anal sphincter, while cats and rabbits predominantly contain type 2 or fast-twitch muscle fibers [21]. The voluntary contraction of external anal sphincter remains at maximum intensity for about 1 minute and then declined to baseline pressure values in about 3 minutes.

Parks and associates found that action potentials are present at rest in patients after spinal cord transection, but were absent in those with tabes dorsalis. These observations show that the muscle tone at rest is regulated by a spinal reflex, in tabes this reflex is interrupted for the destruction of the afferent branch of the spinal reflex [61]. The afferent neurons that activate the reflex have not yet been identified with certainty, but seem likely to be related to receptors relaxation and elongated muscle cells of elevator ani [62].

This hypothesis is confirmed by the observation that rectal distension causes a marked increase in external anal sphincter and pelvic floor (especially muscle puborectal), probably as a result of the tension exerted on muscle receptors.

In proctocolectomy (with ileo-anal anastomosis) muscle tone at rest of the external anal sphincter is not modified in an important way to confirm that the receptors are not in the rectum wall itself but in the context of the sphincter [47,51].

Already Duthie and Gairns, examining multiple histological sections of the rectum, found the presence of sensory endings only in the transitional mucosa of the rectum and anal canal. Receptors pressure and tension in the levator ani and external anal sphincter had been demonstrated previously [63].

On the contrary Ruhl and colleagues demonstrated that sacral dorsal roots contain some afferents from low-threshold mechanoreceptors located in the rectal wall and that these afferents monitor the filling state and the contraction level of the rectum [64,65]. Sensation within the anal canal is carried out by several types of sensory receptors, including free intraepithelial nerve endings (pain), Meissner corpuscles (touch), bulbs of Krause (cold), Pacini corpuscles and Golgi-Mazzoni corpuscles (pressure and tension), and genital corpuscles (friction) [63]. Despite an extensive network of nerves within the anal mucosa, anal continence does not rely heavily on input from these nerve endings. They are thought to play only a minor role in discrimination between the states of fecal matter. Thus, when this area is anesthetized, discrimination between solid and gas is impaired; however, continence is maintained [17,66].

The tonically active puborectalis muscle maintains the resting anorectal angle. Moreover, puborectalis contraction during a sudden rise in abdominal pressure reduces the anorectal angle, preserving continence. While cadaveric studies suggested the puborectalis was supplied by the pudendal nerve, electrophysiological stimulation studies in humans suggested this muscle is supplied, strictly ipsilaterally, by branches originating from the sacral plexus above the pelvic floor. Disruption of the puborectalis inevitably causes significant incontinence, underscoring the importance of this muscle in maintaining continence [21]

Once the rectum is distended, the internal sphincter relaxes (rectoanal inhibitory reflex) and the external sphincter contracts maintaining continence during the period in which the fecal material reaches the anorectal transitional zone where they are thickened sensory receptors. If the distension of the rectum is high, the limit of adaptation, the endorectal pressure reach critical values such as to induce a total inhibition of the sphincter with a sense of urgency to defecation. If the time is right for defecation, the voluntary relaxation of external anal sphincter in combination with other physiological mechanisms enable flushing.

Relaxation of the puborectalis sling produces a widening of the anorectal angle (normally 60-105°, increases to 140°) producing an unobstructed anal pathway which facilitates defecation. Adding the pressure of a Valsalva maneuver overcomes the resistance of the external sphincter and the pelvic floor descends. If the external anal sphincter receives inhibiting signals causing relaxation, the fecal bolus passes. Timing results from the balance of environmental factors acting through cortical inhibition and basic reflexes of the anorectum.

PHYSIOLOGIC TESTING

Multiple techniques have been developed to assess the physiologic function of the pelvic floor, rectum, and sphincters. In conjunction with a detailed history and physical exam, these techniques should be used to assess and detail function, identify and locate a lesion, or solidify a diagnosis. The understanding of many aspects of the physiology of continence and defecation (mechanisms still imperfectly known) uses some instrumental methods such as manometry, electromyography and defecography, nerve stimulation testing, radiographic studies, including endorectal ultrasound and magnetic resonance imaging (MRI).

ANORECTAL MANOMETRY

The anorectal manometry measures pressure in the anal canal to assess the sphincter muscles during rest and voluntary contraction; is the gold standard in diagnosis of functional anorectal disorders. Investigation is crucial in constipation, which often associated with an increase in pressure with a corresponding increase in rectal volumes and capacity, and in the fecal incontinence. Anal manometry becomes an indispensable complement to the morphological investigations, first of all's ultrasound. There is no one standardized method when performing anorectal manometry, and each method has advantages and disadvantages. This method allows detection of:

- baseline pressure profile. Is the evaluation of anal pressure at rest, that value can be obtained by measuring stationary probe to 4-6 channels arranged longitudinally 1 cm away from each other, the expression of the internal anal sphincter tone and allows the calculation of the functional length of the anal canal itself. It is expressed as the maximum pressure in mmHg at rest. The measurement can also be done with extraction at constant speed, a probe at 4-8 channels with radial layout. Using this device allows for a more homogeneous as maintaining constant speed of extraction of the probe.
- dynamic pressure profile. Compared to the previous stage, is to evaluate the pressure in the anal canal starting from 6 up to 1 cm from the anal verge during maximum voluntary contraction. Is defined in this way the maximum pressure reached maximum value as voluntary and its durability, is defined as "squeeze" the difference between maximum pressure and the pressure baseline. This measurement is an index function of the external sphincter, increases lasts for only a minute at most. Squeeze pressure serves only to prevent leakage when the rectal content is presented to the proximal anal canal ad inappropriate times.

- the Rectum Anal Inhibitory Reflex (RAIR) that is evoked through the use of a latex balloon, placed inside rectum and inflated with air. The minimal volume required to elicit the internal anal sphincter relaxation is defined. Normally a testing sequence of 10, 20,30,40 and 50 ml is enough to elicit the RAIR. However, in patients with megarectum much larger volumes may be needed. The internal anal sphincter should normally relax (decrease in pressure 10-15 mmHg) in response to a 30-40 ml balloon distention. The absence of the inhibitory recto-anal reflex for any volume is highly suggestive of Hirschsprung's disease.
- rectal volume sensory thresholds. The first volume of rectal distention that the patient can distinguish to the maximum tolerable volume is determined. Normal values are generally between 100 and 300 ml. Subjects young and constipated patients tend to have greater capacity than rectal elderly and patients with fecal incontinence.
- rectal compliance can be calculated by difference between the volumes of first sensation and maximum tolerable volume divided by the pressure difference ($C = \Delta V / \Delta P$). Rectal compliance refers to the amount of force required to distend the rectal wall. Rectal compliance is measured by inserting an ultrathin polyethylene bag into the rectum. Once in place, the bag is inflated to different volumes, and the pressures from the rectal wall are measured. Multiple measurements are taken and are plotted on a pressure-volume curve. The slope of this curve reflects the compliance of the rectum. There are 3 phases of the compliance curve. The first phase corresponds to the initial resistance and compliance of the rectal wall. The second phase is more compliant as evidenced by the increased volume with pressure changes and represents ''adaptive relaxation'' of the rectal wall. The last phase represents the terminal compliance of the rectal wall and is generally less compliant than the other phases. Urge of defecation occurs during the second phase of compliance. Multiple studies have analyzed the association between anorectal pathologies and rectal compliance findings, and there is still controversy regarding its utility. This technique is also highly variable because of variations in readings of the equipment, variations in patient's physiology, and interobserver variations in readings [17].

Excessive rectal compliance means that a large volume difference corresponds to a small change in pressure with a tendency to rectal bulging. In contrast, a low compliance leads to a significant increase in pressure in response to small volume changes. Compliance, as well as the rectal capacity, varies with age. The normal rectal compliance is

- generally 2-6 ml H2O/mmHg. The normal rectal compliance seems to depend on an intact nervous system and the inherent vitality muscolare.
- the sphincter length can be calculated by performing a stationary / slow or a rapid pull through of the sphincter. The high pressure zone (HPZ) defined as the length of the internal anal sphincter. The length of the HPZ is usually between 2 to 3 cm in women and 2.5 - 3.5 cm in men 1. The HPZ indicates the sphincter length.
- the push / strain maneuver, the external anal sphincter should normally relax during this maneuver
- the average resting tone of the anal canal in healthy adults is generally between 50 and 70 mmHg and is lower in older people without gender differences.
- the maximum resting pressure is usually measured at 1 to 2 cm cranial to anal margin1. The resting pressure in the anal canal is due to 55% - 60% to 3 internal sphincter, 25% - 30% to the external sphincter 4 and the remaining 15% of the maximum pressure at rest in a hemorrhoidal plexus [21].
- vector volume. The pressure profile of the sphincter can also be studied by using a specific catheter with six to eight radially orientated channels; a so-called "vector volume". The vector asymmetry index is calculated considering the total value of all the differences between the pressure of each canal minus the mean value of all pressures. This analysis can give additional information regarding the geometry of the sphincter. Possible deficiencies and asymmetries are shown on a three-dimensional picture. The symmetry of the pressure vectors can be quantified and expressed through an index of asymmetry. Its maximum value in healthy individuals is 10%. Sphincter injury generate a radial pressure gradient with a higher mean asymmetry index of 20% in sleep and contraction [7]. Damon et al have recently shown that an index of asymmetry in HPZ of $\geq$ 25% is related to combined sphincter defects (sensitivity 81% specificity 71%) and that the same index squeeze $\geq$ 25% is related to wide defects of the external sphincter (sensitivity 100% specificity 76%) [67].

Now recognized the undoubted utility of manometry in the diagnosis and treatment choices in the most "common" diseases anorectal new perspectives offers vector study for the best understanding of functional disorders. The three-dimensional vectormanometry allows for an integrated mapping of the radial pressure profiles necessary for identification of pressure asymmetries in the canal anal that, in our experience, are significantly correlated to anal sphincter injures.

In our study, fifty-seven patients, out of 387, complained of fecal incontinence; the rate of asymmetric patients (75,4%) was significantly higher in incontinent group rather than in continent subject (p<0,0001). Also 142/387 (37%) had a rectal prolapse, 55% of patients with rectal prolapse had an asymmetry index >20% and the difference between asymmetric patients rate in presence or in absence of rectal prolapse was statistically significant (p= 0.0446). Finally, 92/387 (24%) was suffering of obstructed defecation, 45,6% of patients of these had an asymmetry index > 20% and the difference between asymmetric patients rate in presence or in absence of obstructed defecation were not statistically significant (p= 0.6004).

Several hypotheses have been suggested to explain this manometric finding such as a pudendal neuropathy or, more likely, a malfunction of the internal anal sphincter due to a sphincter distortion by the prolapse or intussusceptions [68].

In conclusion anal vector manometry, using vector analysis of resting and squeeze anal pressure, and vector asymmetric index scoring are effective tools complementary to anal ultrasonography and provide information on both function and integrity of the anal sphincters. Vector asymmetry index>20% correlates with fecal incontinence due to anal sphincter lesions. Therefore, the anal vector manometry may be useful as an independent method of screening for pregnant women at risk of sphincter injury and for patients undergoing anorectal surgery at risk for incontinence, like previous anorectal surgery or history of two or more previous vaginal deliveries.

Electromyography

Although endoanal ultrasound and MRI have shown superiority over electromyography (EMG) for localization of sphincter defects and elimination of the need for painful probe placement and the need for ionizing radiation, EMG can be used as an alternative technique [17].

Defecography

Defecography can be used to investigate several anorectal abnormalities. It can measure the anorectal angle, the position of the pelvic floor at rest or during Valsalva (perineal descent), the presence of a rectocele, rectal intussusception, and function, including the ability to expel rectal contents.

Ultrasound

Ultrasonography can evaluate anal sphincter integrity and augment manometry and assess anorectal angles and puborectalis function. Ultrasonography evaluates discontinuity in anal sphincters, indicating a prior injury that may be seen in up to 30% of postvaginal deliveries. The internal and external sphincters can be evaluated separately. Various angles are measured with the patient at rest and during maximal voluntary contraction of the puborectalis. Ultrasonography does have the advantage of avoiding exposure to radiation and allows for longer viewing time. Anal ultrasonography relies on the operator for accuracy, but in experienced hands, it can be the mainstay for anal anatomic investigations. In addition, it can provide information regarding the presence and location of anorectal abscess and fistula and staging of tumors [17].

SYMPTOMS AND DIAGNOSIS

In most cases the first symptoms of an anal fissure is an intense pain during defecation with continuous stimulation (tenesmus), accompanied by burning and itching.

The pain may last only a few minutes but also persist for several hours. Classically the pain of the fissure occurs in three different times: the beginning, during the passage of stool is fairly acute, then there is a phase of "stalled", at which time the pain may even disappear altogether, but after a few minutes, come back stronger than ever persist for hours.

These symptoms are known as "pain syndrome in three times of the anal fissure." The pain is both a consequence who cause of spasm. In some cases the pain is so intense that the patients, frightened by defecation, try to avoid it for several days, becoming even more constipated and making it even more painful than the next, inevitable, evacuation.

Sometimes the pain and spastic contraction of the anal sphincter muscles extend to the front of the pelvic floor causing urinary symptoms (pain or difficulty urinating). Usually at the end of defecation may be a slight bleeding which consists of a streak of bright red blood on toilet paper or on the stool.

It is, however, contained hemorrhage that has nothing to do with the most abundant associated with hemorrhoidal disease. Since in some cases the two diseases are associated, the presence of traces of blood may be due to the concomitant presence of hemorrhoids or other injuries.

When the fissure secretes a considerable amount of serum can make the anus "wet" causing itching.

The proctological visit includes accurate medical history, digital exploration of the anal canal and anus-proctoscopy.

The specialist must first rule out other conditions such as hemorrhoids, cancer of the anus and rectum, inflammatory bowel disease, sexually transmitted diseases.

The patient is best placed in the lateral Sims position on a flat table with his right hand retracting the right buttock as an aid to the examiner. The prone position in a "jack-knife" attitude, which offers excellent access to the perineum, requires a special bed proctology.

Is appropriate to take the examination very gently, at first gently widening laterally to the perineal region to deploy the mucocutaneous junction and then put out the fissure, just inside the anus. Often the tear is visible, usually this is all that's needed to diagnose an anal fissure. The research of the anal fissure is facilitated by the presence, at the lower end, hemorrhoid- like thickening of the mucosa, called "sentinel pile."

The rectal examination, when possible for painful, can confirm the site of pain and then the fissure and is also appreciable hypertonia of the sphincter.

The digital examination and proctoscope can cause severe pain with inability to see the ulcer. In this case you will need to take the exam under sedation.

It is advisable to make diagnosis of anal fissure by simple inspection, referring rectal and proctoscopy examinations until the symptoms are not resolved with medical treatment or until surgery to be done under anesthesia.

In the case of fissures refractory to medical therapy or surgery, or in the case of atypical appearance or location biopsy should be made to exclude other diseases such as Crohn's disease, anal cancer or sexually transmitted diseases. In case of bleeding, depending on the chronicity of symptoms, correlation with physical findings, patient's age and the presence or absence of other risk factors for cancer, should be considered the appropriateness of an endoscopic examination of the colon.

Only the anal manometry can confirm the presence of internal sphincter hypertonia. Furthermore, knowing the degree of hypertonia and the length of the sphincter is possible to calibrate the extent of sphincterotomy. Calibrated sphincterotomy may represent an effective and safe procedure for the treatment of chronic anal fissure

REFERENCES

[1] Symington J. The rectum and anus. *J. Anat. Physiol.* 1888; 23: 106-12.
[2] Morgan CN, Thompson HR. Surgical anatomy of the anal canal with special reference to the surgical importance of the internal sphyncter and conjoint longitudinal muscle. *Ann. R. Coll. Surg. Engl.* 1956; 19:88-94.
[3] Goligher J. *Surgery of the anus, rectum and colon.* Bailliere-Tindall, London, 1984.
[4] Kieghley MRB, Williams NS. *Surgery of the anus, rectum and colon.* WB Saunders Company Ltd,London, 1993.
[5] Fielding LP, Goldberg SM. Surgery of the colon, rectum and anus. Butterworth Heinemann Ltd, Oxford, 1993.
[6] Sato K, Sato T. The vascular and neuronal composition of the lateral ligament of the rectum and the rectosacral fascia. *Surg. Radiol. Anat.* 1991; 13: 17-22.
[7] Gordon PH, Nivatvongs S. *Principles and practice of surgery for the colon, rectum and anus.* Quality Medical Publishing Inc, St Louis, 1992.
[8] Fenger C. Histology of the anal canal. *Am. J. Surg. Pathol.* 1988; 12: 41-6.
[9] Fenger C. The anal transitional zone. A method for macroscopic demonstration. *Acta Pathol. Microbiol. Scand.* 1978; 86: 225-32.
[10] Fenger C. The anal transitional zone. *APMIS 1987*; 95 (Suppl 289): 1-9.
[11] Messinetti S, Giacomelli L, Manno A. Il cancro del canale anale. *Utet*, Milano, 1993.
[12] Milligan ETC, Morgan CN. Surgical anatomy of the anal canal with special reference to ano-rectal Fistulae. *Lancet* 1934; ii: 1213-9.
[13] Fenger C. The anal transitional zone. Location and extent. *Acta Pathol. Microbiol. Scand.* 1979; 87: 379-84.
[14] Nivatvongs S, Stern HS, Fryd DS. The lenght or the anal canal. *Dis. colon Rectum* 1982; 24: 600-4.
[15] Bacon HE, Recio PM. *Surgical anatomy of the colon, rectum and anal canal.* Pitmann Medical Publishing Co Ltd JB Lippincott Company, Philadelphia, 1962.
[16] Testut L, Latarjet A. Trattato di anatomia umana. *Utet*, Torino, 1977.
[17] Barleben A., Mills S.: *Anorectal Anatomy and Physiology Surg. Clin. N. Am.* 90 (2010) 1–15
[18] Garavoglia M, Borghi F, Bargoni A, Fronticelli CM. Elementi di sospensione del canale anale. Considerazioni anatomo-chirurgiche. *Minerva Chir.* 1989; 44:1623-31.

[19] Parks AG. The surgical treatment of hemorrhoids. *Br. J. Surg.* 1955; 43: 337-42.
[20] Gold DM, Bartram CI, Halligan S, Kamm MA, Kmiot WA. The quantification of normal anal canal anatomy and sphincter defects using three-dimensional endoanal sonography. *Br. J. Surg.* 1998; 85 (Suppl l): 1.
[21] Bharucha A.E.: Pelvic floor: anatomy and function. *Neurogastroenterol. Motil.* (2006) 18, 507-519
[22] Goligher JC, Leacock AG, Brossy J. The surgical anatomy of the anal canal. *Br. J. Surg.* 1955; 43: 51-23.
[23] Corman ML. Colon and rectal surgery.5th edition. *JB Lippincott*, Philadelphia, 2005.
[24] Stoker J.: Anorectal and pelvic floor anatomy, *Best Practice and Research Clinical Gastroenterology* 23 (2009) 463–475.
[25] Shaflk A. A new concept of the anatomy of the anal sphincter mechanism and the physiology of defecation. III. The longitudinal anal muscle: anatomy and role in anal sphincter mechanism. *Invest. Urol.* 1976; 13: 271-9.
[26] Shafik A, Gamal el-Din MA, el-Sibaei O, Abdel Hamid Z, el-Said B. Involuntary action of the external anal sphincter: manometric and electromyographic studies. *Eur. Surg. Res.* 1992; 24: 188-93.
[27] Garavoglia M, Levi AC, Borghi F, Bargoni A. Considerazioni anatomo-chirurgiche sull'apparato muscolare del canale anale. *Minerva Chir.* 1987; 42:1085-91.
[28] Courtney H. Anatomy of the pelvic diaphragm and anorectal musculature as related to sphincter preservation in anorectal surgery. *Am. J. Surg.* 1950; 79: 155-61.
[29] Garavoglia M, Borghi F, Levi AC. Arrangement of the anal striated musculature. *Dis Colon Rectum* 1993; 36:10-3.
[30] Fowler R. Landmarks and legends of the anal canal. *Aust. N. Z. J. Surg.* 1957; 27:1-6.
[31] Shafik A. A new concept on the anatomy of sphincter mechanism and the physiology of defecation. The external anal sphincter: a triple-loop System. *Invest. Urol.* 1975; 12: 412-8.
[32] Dalley AF. The riddle of the sphincters. The morphophysiology of the anorectal mechanism reviewed. *Am. Surg.* 1987; 53: 298-301
[33] Ayoub SF. Anatomy of the external sphincter in man. *Acta Anat.* 1979; 105:25-31.
[34] Oh C, Kark AE. Anatomy of the external sphincter. *Br. J. Surg.* 1972; 59: 717-721.

[35] Shafik A. A new concept of the anatomy of the anal sphincter mechanism and the physiology of defecation. II. Anatomy of the levator ani muscle with special reference to puborectalis. *Invest. Urol.* 1975; 13:175-82.

[36] Percy JP, Swash M, Neill ME, Parks AG. Electrophysiological study of motor nerve supply of pelvic floor. *Lancet* 1981; ii: 16-20.

[37] Huber A, von Hochstetter A, Allgower M. Anatomy of the pelvic floor for translevatoric-transsphincteric operations. *Am. Surg.* 1987; 53: 247-52.

[38] Shepherd JJ. Anorectal function. In Sircus W, Smith AN, Eds. Scientiflc foundations of gastroenterology. Heinemann, London, 1980.

[39] Shafik A., Asaad S., Doss S.: The histomorphologic structure of the levator ani muscle and its functional significance. *Int. Urogynecol. J.* (2002) 13: 116-124.

[40] Siddhart P, Ravo B. Colorectal neurovasculature and anal sphincter. *Surg. Clin. N. Am.* 1988; 68: 1185-96.

[41] Netter FH. Atlante di anatomia. *Chiba-Geigy*, Varese, 1984.

[42] Patricio J, Bemades A, Nuno D, Falcao F, Silvera L. Surgical anatomy of the arterial blood-supply of the human rectum. *Surg. Radiol. Anat.* 1988; 10: 71-8.

[43] Stelzner F, Staubesand J, Machleidt H. Das corpus cavemosum recti die grundlage der inneren hamorrhoiden. *Langenbecks Arch. Klin. Chr.* 1962; 299:302-306.

[44] Di Matteo G. Principi e tecniche nella chirurgia per cancro del retto sottoperitoneale. *Collana Monografica Società Italiana dì Chinirgia*, Roma, 1995.

[45] Bauer JJ, Gelernt IM, Salky B, et al. Sexual dysfunction following proctocolectomy for benign disease of the colon and rectum. *Ann. Surg.* 1983;197:363–7.

[46] Grigorescu BA, Lazarou G, Olson TR, et al. Innervation of the levator ani muscles: description of the nerve branches to the pubococcygeus, iliococcygeus, and puborectalis muscles. *Int. Urogynecol. J. Pelvic Floor Dysfunct* 2008;19:107–16.

[47] Di Matteo Q. Principi e tecniche nella Chirurgia per cancro del retto sottoperitoneale. *Collana Monografica della Società Italiana di Chirurgia*, Roma, 1995.

[48] Davis K., Kumar D.: Posterior pelvic floor compartment disorders. *Best Pract. Res. Clin. Obstet .Gynaecol.* 2005 Dec;19(6):941-958.

[49] Arhan P, Faverdin C, Persoz B, Devroede G, Dubois F, Domie C. Relationship between viscoelastic properties of the rectum and pressure in man. *J. Appl. Physiol.* 1976; 41: 677-83.

[50] Arhan P, Devroede G, Persoz B, Faverdin C, Dornic C, Pellerin D. Response of the anal canal to repeated distension of the rectum. *Clin. Invest. Med.* 1979;2(2-3):83-8.

[51] Yamada T, Alpers DH, Kaplowitz N, Laine L, Owyang C, Powell DW. *Textbook of gastroenterology.* 4th Edition. (Eds) Lippincott Williams and Wilkins, Philadelphia 2004.

[52] Bennett RC, Duthie HL The functional importance of the internal anal sphincter. *Br. J. Surg.* 1964; 51: 355-9.

[53] Shepherd JJ, Wright PG. The response of internal anal sphincter in man to stimulation of the presacral nerve. *Am. J. Dig. Dis.* 1968; 13: 421-5.

[54] Duthie HL, Watts JM. Contribution of the external anal sphincter to the pressure zone in the anal canal. *Gut.* 1965; 6: 64-8.

[55] Penninckx F., Lestar B., Kerremans R.: The internal anal sphincter: mechanisms of control and its role in maintaining anal continence. *Baillieres Clin. Gastroenterol.* (1992) 6: 193-214.

[56] Duthie GS, Bartolo DC. Faecal continence and defecation. In *coloproctology and the pelvic floor*. Butterworth-Heinemann, Oxford, 1992.

[57] Burleigh DE, D'Mello A. Physiology and pharmacology of the internal anal sphincter. In Henry MM, Swash M, Eds. *Coloproctology and pelvic floor*. Butterworths, London, 1985.

[58] .Mathers S. Neural control of the pelvic sphincters. *In coloproctology and the pelvic floor*. Butterworth-Heinemann, Oxford, 1992.

[59] Freukner B, von Euler C. Influence of pudendal nerve block on the function of the anal sphincters. *Gut.* 1975; 16: 482-5.

[60] Pency JP, Neill ME, Swash M, Parte AG. Electrophysiological study of motor nerve supply of pelvic floor. *Lancet* 1981; i: 16-9.

[61] Parks AG, Porter NH, Melzak J. Experimental study of the reflex mechanism controlling the muscles of the pelvic floor. *Dis. Colon Rectum* 1962; 5: 407-11.

[62] Phillips SF, Edwards D. Some aspects of anal continence and defecation. *Gut.* 1965; 6: 396-401.

[63] Duthie HL, Gains FW. Sensory ending and sensation in the anal region of man. *Br. J. Surg.* 1960; 47: 585-9.

[64] Ruhl A, Thewissen M, Ross HG, et al. Discharge patterns of intramural mechanoreceptive afferents during selective distension of the cat's rectum. *Neurogastroenterol. Motil.* 1998;10:219–25.

[65] Gowers WR. The automatic action of the sphincter ani. *Proc. R. Soc. Lond* 1877;26: 77-82.

[66] Cherry DA, Rothenberger DA. Pelvic floor physiology. *Surg. Clin. North Am.* 1988; 68:1217–30.
[67] Mounier P, Mollard P. Control of the internal anal sphincter (manometric study with human subjects). *Pflugers Archiv.* 1977; 370: 233-9.
[68] Damon H, Henry L, Roman S, Barth X, Mion F: Influence of rectal prolapsed on the asymmetry of the anal sphincter in patients with anal incontinence. *BMC Gastroenterol* 2003; 19: 3-23.

In: Anal Fissure
Editors: P. Sileri and A. L. Gaspari

ISBN: 978-1-61209-716-9
© 2012 Nova Science Publishers, Inc

Chapter 2

CHEMICAL SPHINCTEROTOMY

Giovanni Milito and Federica Cadeddu
The Department of Surgery, University Hospital Tor Vergata, Rome, Italy

ABSTRACT

Although the debate about optimum first-line therapy for chronic fissure continues, treatment is becoming increasingly medical.

Chemical sphincterotomy is effective in decreasing symptoms, improving healing of chronic anal fissure and avoiding the risk of anal incontinence associated with surgical treatment. Glyceryl trinitrate, a nitric oxide donor, is the first medical agent used and is now a well established first-line treatment.

However, some authors reported an high incidence of side effects with glyceryl trinitrate, particularly a severe headache in over 30% of patients, forcing some subjects to stop the treatment.

Twice-daily application of 0.2 percent glyceryl trinitrate ointment and, besides, local application of calcium channel blockers to the distal anal canal and anal margin lowers anal resting pressure, increases local blood flow, decrease anal pain leading to fissure healing in over two thirds of patients according to some authors.

Alternative medical therapies including α1-adrenoceptor antagonists (indoramin) cholinergic agonists (bethanechol) endogenous nitric oxide donors(L-arginine), and phosphodiesterase Inhibitors are being tested in an effort to avoid the side effects of nitroglicerine but remain at a developmental stage.

All these non surgical treatments are discussed in the present chapter with a focus on chemical composition and mechanism of action of these agents, safety profile and surgical results reported in literature.

INTRODUCTION

Greater than 90% of acute anal fissures are of short duration and heal spontaneously or with simple measures. A high-fiber diet with an increased intake of water is recommended, laxatives may be used when required to soften constipated stool and warm sitz baths may offer symptomatic relief. Acute fissures that fail to heal become chronic fissures, which have traditionally been treated by surgery [1].

Chronicity is defined by both chronology and morphology. Most surgeons consider the persistence for 6 weeks as a reasonable cut-off to define a chronic anal fissure. Morphologically, chronic anal fissure is characterized by the presence of 1.visible transverse IAS fibers at the bottom of a fissure; 2. indurated edges; 3. sentinel pile 4. hypertropical anal papilla [2].

The presence of an anal fissure is reliably associated with an elevated intra-anal pressure and decreased blood flow to the anoderm. The increased pressure is generated by hypertonicity of the internal anal sphincter that includes blood vessels to the anoderm. The main target of the treatment of anal fissure is the IAS spasm reduction, either by pharmacologic agents or performing sphincterotomy [1,2].

Traditionally, lateral internal sphincterotomy has been considered the gold standard treatment for chronic fissures, but this procedure requires anaesthesia and is associated with a noteworthy risk of incontinence. More recently, various pharmacologic agents have been shown to decrease resting anal pressure and promote fissure healing. This so-called *chemical sphincterotomy* has been used as first-line treatment for chronic anal fissure in many centres [1,3].

Chemical sphincterotomy is particularly suitable in presence of risk factors for incontinence (previous anorectal surgery, history of multiple vaginal deliveries, prior incontinence, inflammatory bowel diseases) when sphincterotomy for anal fissure generally has an additional risk. In case of pharmacologic therapy failure or fissures recurrence, when patients have high resting anal pressure, lateral internal sphincterotomy is the treatment of choice [3].

Topical 0.2% GTN ointment has been the first chemical agent used in clinical practice[4]. Subsequently other drugs have shown effective results with fewer side effects; an important advantage of these novel treatments is that by acting through different pathways, they may be effective in the 30% of cases in which GTN fails.

NITRATES

In the gastrointestinal tract, NO mediates NANC evoked relaxation of the longitudinal and circular smooth muscle from the lower oesophageal sphincter, stomach, duodenum, small intestine and internal anal sphincter [5]. Loder *et al* [6] and Guillemot *et al.* [7,8] demonstrated that topically applied NTG causes a significant reduction in resting anal canal pressure of normal human beings.

The recognition of nitric oxide as a neurotransmitter mediating relaxation of the internal anal sphincter (figures 1 and 2) led to the widespread use of organic nitrates in the treatment of chronic anal fissure [9].

Preparations of isosorbide dinitrate and GTN have been effective to treat chronic anal fissure. The proposed mechanism of action has been reduced anal sphincter pressure or a primary or secondary increase in anal blood flow.

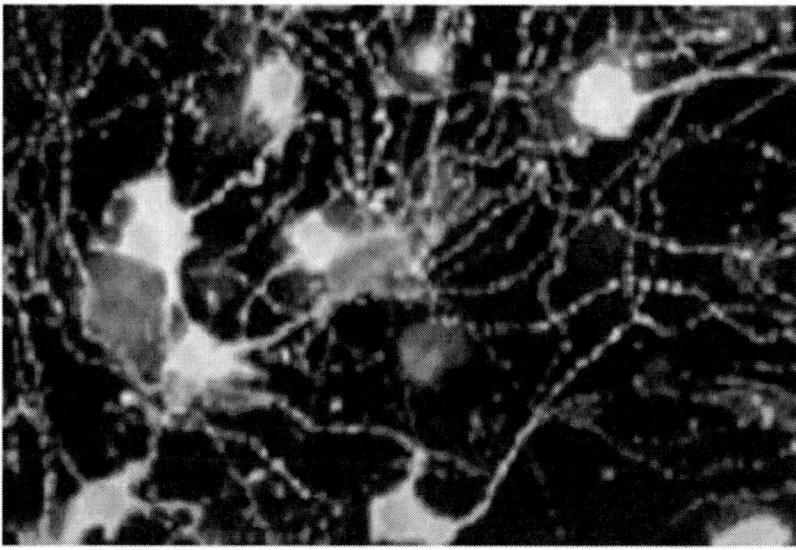

Figure 1. NO neurons included in the myenteric plexus of the bowel.

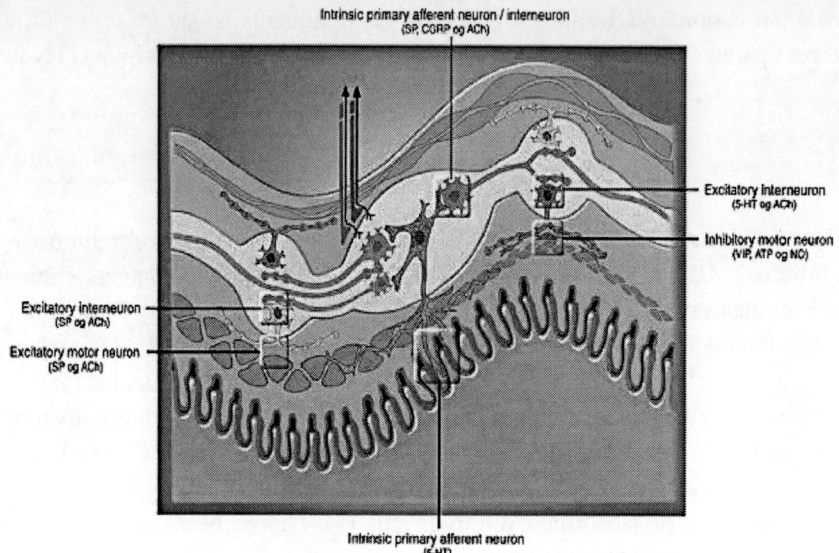

Figure 2. Pathways of the enteric nervous system: NO motor neurons inhibits muscle contraction.

GTN and isosorbide dinitrate act as nitric oxide donors, being metabolized at a cellular level to release this compound. In these situations NO evokes a membrane hyperpolarization. NANC-stimulated relaxation of gastrointestinal smooth muscle is associated with an initial rapid hyperpolarization (large amplitude) followed by a sustained hyperpolarization (small amplitude). NO appears to mediate the latter hyperpolarization.

Nitric oxide mediates relaxation of the internal sphincter through the guanylyl cyclase pathway by increasing cyclic guanosine monophosphate levels within the smooth muscle cells [5,9].

Organic nitrates chemically represent esters of nitric acid (HNO3) with mono- or polyhydric alcohols. Individual potency of organic nitrates is proportional to the number of nitrate groups per molecule and is a function of their lipophility. Organic nitrates differ in their pharmacokinetics from each other. GTN is eliminated at a much faster rate than isosorbide mononitrate but, despite this, steady state concentrations of GTN can be maintained by transdermal formulations. When applied as an ointment, the absorption amount usually exceeds skin permeability that determines how much drug reaches the plasma. Thus, variable skin permeability, difficulty in standardizing the surface area and continuous changes in concentration gradient between ointment and plasma, lead to irregular absorption and fluctuating plasma concentrations of GTN and isosorbide dinitrate [11,12].

Several studies have investigated the effect of topical glyceryl trinitrate ointment and supported the use of 0.2 to 0.4 percent nitroglycerin ointment for the treatment of anal fissure. Healing rates range from 30% to 86% [13](chart 1).

Chart 1. Results in literature of gliceril trinitrate for the treatment of chronic anal fissure

Authors, year	Patients N	Agent	Healing rate %	Headache %
Loder et al, 1994[6]	20	0,2 % GTN	NR	10
Oettlé, 1997[28]	12		83	0
Lund and Scholefield, 1997[14]	38	0,2 % GTN	68	58
Carapeti et al, 1999[16]	23	0,2 % GTN	65	72
Brisinda et al, 1999[25]	25	0,2 % GTN	60	20
Kennedy et al, 1999[15]	43	0,2 % GTN	46	NR
Zuberi et al, 2000[17]	18	0,2 % GTN	67	72
Altomare et, al, 2000[19]	59	0,2 % GTN	49	34
Richards et al 2000[32]	44	0,2 % GTN*	29.5	20.5
Pitt et al, 2001[20]	64	0,2 % GTN	41	64
Bailey et al, 2002[22]	304	0,0.1,0.2,0.4% GTN	50	
Mishra et al, 2005[30]	20	0,2 % GTN*	30 at 4 weeks	NR
Brown CJ et al, 2007[34]	27	0,2 % GTN*	56	NR
Brisinda et al, 2007[26]	50	0.2% GTN	70	34
Sileri et al, 2010[35]	311	0.2% GTN or AD	54.5 at 12 weeks	

*Randomized trial GTN versus lateral internal sphincterotomy; GTN gliceril trinitrate; NR not reported; AD anal dilatators.

Recently, Lund randomized 80 patients to 0.2 per cent GTN (twice daily for 8 weeks) or to placebo paste [14]. Healing rates were significantly higher in the GTN group (68 *versus* 8 per cent; $P < 0.001$), but headaches were common (58 *versus* 18 per cent). Differently, Kennedy et al [15] reported an healing rate of 46% in the GNT group versus 16% in the placebo arm. In the longer term, 35 per cent of patients were submitted to internal sphincterotomy.

Carapeti *et al* [16] from St Mark's Hospital randomized 70 patients to GTN or placebo using higher doses of GTN (three times daily for 8 weeks). After eight weeks fissure had healed in 67% of patients treated with GTN compared with 32% with placebo (p=0.008). Neither improvement of results nor increase of morbidity were detected.

Recently Zuberi et al [17] compared GTN patches applied to the buttocks to topical 0.2% GTN and surgery in a randomized study. Forty-two consecutive patients with chronic anal fissure were randomized to 0.2% GTN ointment or 10-mg nitroglycerin patch for 8 weeks and a 12 controls underwent surgery without significant difference in healing rate.

Although the initial results of GNT treatment were promising, subsequently concerns over medium-term relapse, tachyphylaxis and morbidity have been raised [13, 18].

In a multicentre randomized Italian trial on 132 patients, Altomare, Milito and coworkers [19] failed to demonstrate the superiority of GTN (twice daily for 4 weeks) over placebo (49 *versus* 52 per cent). Besides, improvements in pain and anodermal blood flow, as well as a reduction in resting pressure, were demonstrated.

Different studies have suggested explanations for the poor healing rates with GTN. In a recent retrospective trial Pitt reported an healing rate of 41% and a relapse rate of 50% in 64 patients 52. Two independent risk factors for failure to heal were found: the presence of a sentinel pile *(P < 0.035)* and a history of fissure longer than 6 months *(P < 0,019)*[20].

Furthermore, direct comparison of trials is complicated by heterogeneity of the topical preparations, different dosages and duration of treatment, selection criteria for chronic anal fissures, and the duration of symptoms before treatment.

Recently Azarnoff et al [21] evaluated the quality of nitrate preparations and found that over 40% of samples analyzed did not meet the United States Pharmacopoeia specifications for potency and/or content uniformity when filling a prescription for 0.3 percent nitroglycerin ointment. Subpotent nitroglycerin ointment and/or not uniformly distributed nitroglycerin throughout the product are much less likely to relieve patients anal fissure pain, a severe and debilitating symptom that may affect their ability to work.

In a randomized multicenter trial of ASCRS, Bailey et al [22] tried to find the optimal treatment schedule of GNT to achieve fissure healing. A randomized, double- blind study of intra-anally applied nitroglycerin ointment (Anogesic™) was conducted in 304 patients randomized to 0.0, 0.1, 0.2, 0.4 percent nitroglycerin ointment applied twice or three times per day up to eight weeks. Nitroglycerin ointment significantly and rapidly reduced the pain associated with chronic anal fissures; a 0.4% concentration (1.5 mg GTN) was the most effective. The healing rate was approximately 50 percent in each group including placebo.

The most common side effects of nitrates are headache and hypotension. The incidence of moderate to severe headaches is up to 84% of patients. Headache is particularly evident at higher concentrations of the drug. Compliance can be improved if the patients are warned of headache as a side effect and told that it is often easily dealt with by simple analgesia before application of the ointment. However, compliance seems not to be significantly affected by headache and treatment drop-outs are uncommon [23, 24].

Anal burning as a result of treatment with nitroglycerin has also been reported [13]. There is a potential for methaemoglobinaemia but this side effect is rare after clinical doses. In some patients, abrupt withdrawal of nitrates may bring about rebound responses in several haemodynamic parameters.

NITRATES VERSUS BOTULINUM TOXIN

Since their introduction nitrates have been compared to surgical and medical agents in the treatment of chronic anal fissure. Botulinum toxin injection into anal sphincter is another therapeutic approach which have been used to treat chronic anal fissure and avoid the risk of permanent injury to the anal sphincter.

In a study by Brisinda *et al* [25], 50 patients were randomized to receive 20 U of Botox, administered as two injections on each side of the anterior midline of the internal sphincter, or 0.2% nitroglycerine ointment. After 2 months, the fissures were healed in 24 of 25 patients (96%) in the botulinum toxin group and 15 of 25 patients (60%) in the GTN group. No patient in either group had fecal incontinence or suffered from relapse. Similarly, in a following larger experience, the authors randomized 100 adults to receive treatment with either type A botulinum toxin — 30 units Botox® or 90 units Dysport® — injected into the internal anal sphincter or 0.2 percent nitroglycerin ointment applied three times daily for eight weeks. After two months, healing rate in botulinum arm was 92 percent versus 70 percent in the nitroglycerin group (P =0.009). Twenty patients — 3 in the botulinum toxin group and 17 in the nitroglycerin group (P <0.001) — reported adverse effects: mild transient incontinence of flatus in botulinum group and moderate-to-severe headache in the nitroglycerin arm [26].

In a recent study with 30 patients, Lysy *et al.* compared the therapeutic effect of botulinum toxin injection plus local application of isosorbide dinitrate (group A) with botulinum toxin given alone (group B). At 6 wk, the fissure healing rate was significantly higher in group A compared with group B (66% vs 20%). Nevertheless, at 8 and 12 wk, no significant differences were seen [27].

NITRATES VERSUS ANAL SPHINCTEROTOMY

The first small clinical experience comparing nitrates and sphincterotomy was conducted by Oettlé et al who randomized 24 patients to topical GTN or LIS for chronic anal fissure treatment 28. Although only 83% of patients using GTN healed compared to 100% in the surgical group, the difference was not statistically significant ($p=0.239$).

Subsequently larger randomized trials showed a higher efficacy of surgical treatment compared to nitrates [29, 30].

Evans et al [31] randomized 59 patients to 0.2 percent GTN three times a day for eight weeks or to LIS. Twenty of 33 (60.6 percent) glyceryl trinitrate patients had healed fissures in eight weeks compared with 26 of 27 (97 percent) in the sphincterotomy group (P = 0.001). Poor tolerance and poor compliance with treatment were important factors in patients whose fissures did not heal with glyceryl trinitrate. Similarly, Richards and coworkers [32] randomized patients with symptomatic chronic anal fissures to 0.25 percent nitroglycerin tid (44 pts) or internal sphincterotomy (38 pts). Healing rate was 89.5% in the surgical group versus 29.5% in the nitrates arm.

Parellada et al [33] compared lateral internal sphincterotomy with local 0.2 percent isosorbide dinitrate to treat 54 patients with chronic anal fissure. In nitrate group, healing rate at 10 weeks was 89% versus 100 percent in the surgical arm. Eight patients (30 percent) had minor side effects after ointment versus 44% of minor temporary incontinence after surgery.

Brown and colleagues [34] evaluated the long term outcomes in 82 patients who had participated in a randomized, controlled trial comparing 0.25 percent topical nitroglycerin and lateral internal sphincterotomy. After six years of follow-up, lateral internal sphincterotomy appeared a more durable treatment for chronic anal fissure compared with topical nitroglycerin therapy and does not compromise long-term faecal continence.

In a recent large prospective study Sileri and coworkers treated 311 patients, presenting with chronic anal fissure, with 0.2% nitroglycerin ointment or anal dilators for 8 weeks. If no improvement was observed after 8 weeks, the patients were assigned to the other treatment or a combination of the two. In case of failure after 12 weeks the patients were submitted to botulinum toxin injection into the internal sphincter and fissurectomy or lateral internal sphincterotomy. Overall healing rates were 64.6% and 94% after GTN/DIL or BTX/LIS. Healing rate after BTX was 83.3% and overall healing after LIS group was 98.7% with no definitive incontinence [35].

CALCIUM CHANNEL BLOCKERS

Calcium antagonists prevent the influx of calcium into the smooth muscle cell, decreasing intracellular calcium concentration. This reduces the amount of calcium available to combine with calmodulin and subsequently prevents activation of the myosin light chain kinase required for smooth muscle cell contraction [9, 36].

In 1987 it was showed that anal resting pressure decreased shortly after oral administration of 60 mg diltiazem [37]. More recently, two calcium channel blockers, nifedipine and diltiazem, have been used topically with good healing rate [38, 39] (chart 2).

Chart 2. Results in literature of calcium channel blockers for the treatment of chronic anal fissure

Author, year	Patients N	Agent	Dose	Healing rate %
Antropoli et al 1999[42]	141	Nifedipine	2% ointment	95
Jonas & Scholefield, 2000[58]	24	Diltiazem	60 mg oral	38
Jonas & Scholefield, 2000[58]	26	Diltiazem	2% ointment	65
Carapeti et al. 2000[36]	15	Diltiazem	2% ointment	67
Knight et al, 2001[41]	71	Diltiazem	2% ointment	75
Jonas & Scholefield, 2002[38]	39	Diltiazem	2% ointment	58
Das Gupta et al. 2002[39]	23	Diltiazem	2% ointment	48

In a trial on 47 patients, Griffin et al[40] demonstrated that 2% diltiazem cream was effective in healing approximately 50% of chronic anal fissures that have failed a trial of 0.2% GTN ointment. The incidence of side-effects was minimal (compared to GTN); 45% of patients in this study complained of headaches with the initial course of topical GTN. In a larger study on 72 patients, Knight and coworkers observed a 75% healing rate after treatment with 2% diltiazem ointment [41].

Recently, Antropoli reported a 95% healing rate three weeks after treatment with 0.2% nifedipine gel applied twice compared to only 50% of those in the placebo group ($p<0.01$) with no systemic or local side effects [42].

Different studies have compared the effectiveness of calcium antagonists and of other medical and surgical therapies. In a prospective randomized controlled trial on ninety patients, 2% diltiazem ointment and 0.2% GTN ointment were compared. Diltiazem ointment was found to be superior regarding pain relief, fewer side effects, and late recurrence as compared with GTN ointment [43].

Subsequently, Ho and coworkers randomized 132 patients to lateral internal sphincterotomy, tailored sphincterotomy or oral nifedipine. Surgery was associated with significantly better fissure healing rates ($P < 0.001$ at 16 weeks) and less recurrence ($P = 0.003$) than nifedipine. There were substantial problems with compliance in the nifedipine group (17 of 41 patients), related to side-effects and slow healing [44].

Oral preparations were also effective, but side effects such as headache and flushing were very common and limited their use [9]. Oral nifedipine (Adalat Retard^{TM}; Bayer Pharmaceuticals, Newbury, UK), 20 mg twice daily, produced a 36 per cent fall in MRP in a small open-label study. Healing rates were equivalent to those of GTN (60 per cent); headaches (33 per cent) and flushing (66 per cent) were very common [45].

Recently Ansaloni et al found that lacidipine, given orally in single daily dosage of 6 mg, was associated to an healing rate of 90% at the 28-day follow-up. Unlike most of the other calcium antagonists, including nifedipine, that have a relatively short duration of action and need to be administered 2–3 times daily, lacidipine is a calcium antagonist with a long duration of action, allowing a once-daily administration and besides, is better tolerated than other calcium antagonists [46].

L-ARGININE

Recently, it has been shown in healthy volunteers that L-arginine, being an intrinsic precursor of nitric oxide, reduces anal resting pressure without headache and it induces fissure healing [47]. Subsequently in the phase II trial Gosselink and co-workers treated 15 patients for at least 12 weeks by local application of a gel containing L-arginine 400 mg/ml five times a day after nitrates treatment failure. In patients with a persistent fissure, treatment was continued until 18 weeks. Complete fissure healing was observed in 3 of 13 (23 percent) patients, and after 18 weeks the healing rate was 8 of 13 (62 percent) patients. None of the 13 patients experienced typical nitric oxide-induced headache.

Therefore L-arginine seems effective in patients not responding to isosorbide dinitrate treatment, but larger studies are needed before it can be used as a possible alternative treatment [48].

POTASSIUM CHANNEL OPENERS

Potassium channel openers are effective in smooth muscle relaxation and they are used to treat hypertension. Lignocaine gel is reported as the current medical treatment for chronic anal fissure in South Asian population [9]. In a prospective, double blinded, randomized controlled trial on 50 patients, Ahmad compared topical lignocaine and 0.2% GNT ointment showing that topical GTN has earlier and a higher rate of clinical healing of anal fissure with acceptable side effects and comparable recurrence rate. Symptomatic relief was earlier with GTN as compared with lignocaine. Pain relief was steady and sustained in GTN group. Further, at 8 weeks follow up, 80% of GNT patients showed clinical signs of healing compared to 32% in Group B (p=0.001). Headache was the main side effect of GTN. At 6-month follow-up, recurrence was seen in 3/8 lignoocaine patients compared to 8/20 in the GTN Group (p=1) [49].

These agents seem promising but larger studies are needed before they can be used as a possible alternative treatment. In addition some authors reported development of anal ulceration, in patients treated with nicorandil for symptomatic control of ischaemic heart disease [50, 51]. All ulcers healed after withdrawal of nicorandil. This side effect needs to be clarified.

ALPHA-ADRENOCEPTOR ANTAGONISTS

Anal resting tone and internal anal sphincter activity is enhanced by sympathetic excitatory stimulation via α-adrenoceptors. As a consequence, α-1 adrenoceptor blockade has been proposed as another modality of chemical sphincterotomy [52]. In a preliminary study, Pitt *et al.* assessed the effect of a single oral 20-mg dose of indoramin, an α-adrenoceptor antagonist, in seven patients with chronic anal fissures and in six healthy volunteers [52]. In both groups, indoramin reduced anal resting pressure by a mean of >35%. Treatment with α-adrenoceptor antagonists is still at a developmental stage and currently is not advocated in the treatment of chronic anal fissure.

PHOSPHODIESTERASE-5 INHIBITORS

Phosphodiesterase, the enzyme involved in degradation of cyclic nucleotides, contains a number of different isoenzymes. PDE-5 is primarily located in smooth muscle and is integral to the degradation of cGMP. Sildenafil, a PDE-5 inhibitor, produces inhibition of PDE-5 more selectively han other isoenzymes, resulting in increased intracellular concentrations of cGMP and smooth muscle relaxation [53].

Recently Torrabadella [54] treated 19 patinets with Topical administration of 10 percent sildenafil and reported a 18% reduction in anal sphincter pressure in less than 3 minutes. However further investigation are warranted to clarify the efficacy and safety of these therapeutical agents.

ANGIOTENSIN-CONVERTING ENZYME INHIBITORS

Earlier studies in the IAS have demonstrated the presence of Angiotensin II and AT1 receptors in the internal anal sphincter; thus the renin-angiotensin system might have a role in the modulation of internal anal sphincter tone [55, 56].

Recently, topical captopril (0.28%), an ACE inhibitor, was shown to reduce mean anal resting pressure and maximum resting pressure in 50% of healthy volunteers by up to 44% at 20 minutes [57]. These results are promising, however further investigation are warranted to clarify the effectiveness of this therapeutical agent.

CONCLUSION

Lateral internal sphincterotomy has been considered, over the last century, the most effective treatment to eliminate internal anal sphincter spasm constantly associated to anal fissure, allowing the ulcer to heal. Nevertheless, debate exists regarding the safety of anal sphincterotomy and the controversial risk of incontinence of surgical sphincterotomy has sparked interest in pharmacologic approaches to produce reversible reduction of sphincter pressure and obtain fissure healing minimizing incontinence risk. Glyceryl trinitrate is the first medical agent used and is now a well established first-line treatment.

For topical treatment with GTN, healing rates from 33% to 86% were observed; however, it is associated to severe headache in over two thirds of patients.

In an effort to avoid the side effects of GTN, other medical agents have been proposed. Local application of calcium channel blockers to the distal anal canal and anal margin lowers anal resting pressure, increases local blood flow, decrease anal pain leading to fissure healing in over two thirds of patients according to some authors.

Other approaches such as α1-adrenoceptor antagonists (indoramin) cholinergic agonists (bethanechol) endogenous nitric oxide donors (L-arginine), and phosphodiesterase Inhibitors are still to be examined.

REFERENCES

[1] Madoff, R.D. & Fleshman, J.W. (2003). AGA technical review on the diagnosis and care of patients with anal fissure. *Gastroenterology, 124*, 235-45.

[2] Jonas M. & Scholefield J.H. (2001) Anal fissure. *Gastroenterol. Clin. North Am. 30*:167–181.

[3] Nelson R. (2004) A systematic review of medical therapy for anal fissure. *Dis. Colon. Rectum,47*, 422-31.

[4] Lund J.N. & Scholefield J.H. (1997) Glyceryl trinitrate is an effective treatment for anal fissure. *Dis. Colon Rectum,40*, 468-70.

[5] Davies M.G. Fulton G.J. Hagen P.O. (1995) Clinical biology of nitric oxide. *Br. J. Surg.,82*,1598–1610.

[6] Loder P.B. Kamm M.A. Nicholls R.J. Phillips R.K. (1994) 'Reversible chemical sphincterotomy' by local application of glyceryl trinitrate. *Br. J. Surg.,81*,1386–1389.

[7] Guillemot F. Lone Y.C. Leroi H. Lamblin M.D. Cortot A. (1992) Nitroglycerin in situ reduces upper anal canal pressure. *Dig. Dis. Sci. 37*:155.

[8] Guillemot F. Leroi H. Lone Y.C. Rousseau C.G. Lamblin M.D. Cortot A. (1993) Action of in situ nitroglycerin on upper anal canal pressure of patients with terminal constipation. A pilot study. *Dis. Colon Rectum, 36*,372–376.

[9] Collins E.E &.Lund J.N. (2007) A review of chronic anal fissure management. *Tech. Coloproctol.,11*,209–223.

[10] Fung H.L. (1992) Do nitrates differ? *Br. J. Clin. Pharmacol.,34*,5S–9S.

[11] Bogaert M.G. (1987) Clinical pharmacokinetics of glyceryl trinitrate following the use of systemic and topical preparations. *Clin. Pharmacokinet.,12,*1–11.

[12] Jonas M. Barrett D.A. Shaw P.N. Scholefield J.H. (2001) Systemic levels of glyceryl trinitrate following topical application to the anoderm do not correlate with the measured reduction in anal pressure. *Br. J. Surg., 88*,1613–1616.

[13] Lindsey I. Jones O.M. Cunningham C. Mortensen N.J. (2004) Chronic anal fissure. *Br. J. Surg.,91,*270-9.

[14] Lund J.N. Scholefield J.H.(1997) A randomised, prospective, double-blind, placebo-controlled trial of glyceryl trinitrate ointment in treatment of anal fissure. *Lancet,349*,11-4.

[15] Kennedy M.L. Sowter S. Nguyen H. Lubowski D.Z. (1999) Glyceryl trinitrate ointment for the treatment of chronic anal fissure: results of a placebo-controlled trial and long-term follow-up. *Dis. Colon Rectum, 42*,1000–1006.

[16] Carapeti E.A. Kamm M.A. McDonald P.J. Chadwick S.J.D. Melville D. Phillips R.K.S. (1999) Randomised controlled trial shows that glyceryl trinitrate heals anal fissures, higher doses are not more effective, and there is a high recurrence rate. *Gut., 44*,727–730.

[17] Zuberi B.F. Rajput M.R. Abro H. Shaikh S.A. (2000) A randomized trial of glyceryl trinitrate ointment and nitroglycerin patch in healing of anal fissures. *Int. J. Colorectal. Dis.,15*,243–245.

[18] Nelson R. (2006) Non surgical therapy for anal fissure. *Cochrane Database Syst. Rev.:CD003431*.

[19] Altomare D.F. Rinaldi M., Milito G. et al (2000) Glyceryl trinitrate for chronic anal fissure—healing or headache? Results of a multicenter, randomized, placebo-controled, double-blind trial. *Dis. Colon Rectum, 43*,174–179.

[20] Pitt J. Williams S. Dawson P.M. (2001) Reasons for failure of glyceryl trinitrate treatment of chronic fissure-in-ano: a multivariate analysis. *Dis. Colon. Rectum. ,44*,864–867.

[21] Azarnoff D.L. Lee J.C. Lee C. Chandler J. Karlin D. (2007) Quality of extemporaneously compounded nitroglycerin ointment. *Dis. Colon Rectum, 50*,509–516.

[22] Bailey H.R. Beck D.E. Billingham R.P. et al (2002) A study to determine the nitroglycerin ointment dose and dosing interval that best promote the healing of chronic anal fissures. *Dis. Colon Rectum,45*,1192–1199.
[23] Shah V. Lyford G. Gores G. Farrugia G. (2004) Nitric oxide in gastrointestinal health and disease. *Gastroenterology,126*,903-13.
[24] Salgado G. Torrbedella L. Berman I.R.(1999) Headaches in the treatment of anal fissure. *Dis.Colon Rectum, 42*,1106.
[25] Brisinda G, Maria G, Bentivoglio AR, Cassetta E, Gui D, Albanese A. (1999) A comparison of injections of botulinum toxin and topical nitroglycerin ointment for the treatment of chronic anal fissure. *N. Engl. J. Med.,341*,65-69.
[26] Brisinda G. Cadeddu F. Brandara F. Marniga G. Maria G. (2007) Randomized clinical trial comparing botulinum toxin injections with 0.2 percent nitroglycerin ointment for chronic anal fissure. *British Journal of Surgery,94,*162-167.
[27] Lysy J. Israelit-Yatzkan Y. Sestiery-Ittah M. Weksler-Zangen S. Keret D. Goldin E. (2001) Topical nitrates potentiate the effect of botulinum toxin in the treatment of patients with refractory anal fissure. *Gut.,48*,221-4.
[28] Oettle GJ. (1997) Glyceryl trinitrate vs. sphincterotomy for treatment of chronic fissure-in-ano: a randomized, controlled trial. *Dis. Colon Rectum, 40*,1318–1320.
[29] Libertiny G. Knight JS. Farouk R (2002) Randomised trial of topical 0.2% glyceryl trinitrate and lateral internal sphincterotomy for the treatment of patients with chronic anal fissure: long-term follow-up. *Eur. J. Surg., 168*,418–421.
[30] Mishra R. Thomas S. Maan MS. Hadke NS. (2005) Topical nitroglycerin versus lateral internal sphincterotomy for chronic anal fissure: prospective, randomized trial. *ANZ J. Surg.,75*,1032–1035.
[31] Evans J. Luck A. Hewett P. (2001) Glyceryl trinitrate vs. lateral sphincterotomy for chronic anal fissure: prospective, randomized trial. *Dis. Colon Rectum,44*,93–97.
[32] Richard CS. Gregoire R. Plewes EA. et al (2000) Internal sphincterotomy is superior to topical nitroglycerin in the treatment of chronic anal fissure: results of a randomized, controlled trial by the Canadian Colorectal Surgical Trials Group. *Dis. Colon Rectum,43*,1048–1057.
[33] Parellada C. (2004) Randomized, prospective trial comparing 0.2 percent isosorbide dinitrate ointment with sphincterotomy in treatment of chronic anal fissure: a two-year follow-up. *Dis. Colon Rectum,47*,437–443.

[34] Brown C.J. Dubreuil D. Santoro L. Liu M. O'Connor B.I. McLeod R.S. (2007) Lateral internal sphincterotomy is superior to topical nitroglycerin for healing chronic anal fissure and does not compromise long-term fecal continence: six-year follow-up of a multicenter, randomized, controlled trial. *Dis. Colon Rectum,50*,442–44.

[35] Sileri P. Stolfi V.M. Franceschilli L. Grande M. Di Giorgio A. D'Ugo S. Attina' G. D'Eletto M. Gaspari A.L. (2010) Conservative and surgical treatment of chronic anal fissure: prospective longer term results *J. Gastrointest. Surg.,14*,773-80.

[36] Carapeti EA. Kamm M.A. Phillips R.K. (2000) Topical diltiazem and bethanechol decrease anal sphincter pressure and heal anal fissures without side effects. *Dis. Colon Rectum,43,*1359–1362.

[37] Jonard P. Essamri B. (1987) Diltiazem and internal anal sphincter. *Lancet, 1*,754.

[38] Jonas M. Speake W. Scholefield J.H. (2002) Diltiazem heals glyceryl trinitrate-resistant chronic anal fissures: a prospective study. *Dis. Colon Rectum, 45,*1091–1095.

[39] DasGupta R. Franklin I. Pitt J. Dawson P.M. (2002) Successful treatment of chronic anal fissure with diltiazem gel. *Colorectal. Dis.,4*,20–22.

[40] Griffin N. Acheson A.G. Jonas M. Scholefield J.H. (2002) The role of topical diltiazem in the treatment of chronic anal fissures that have failed glyceryl trinitrate therapy. *Colorectal. Dis.,4*,430–435.

[41] Knight JS. Birks M. Farouk R. (2001) Topical diltiazem ointment in the treatment of chronic anal fissure. *Br. J. Surg.,88*,553–556

[42] Antropoli C. Perrotti P. Rubino M. et al (1999) Nifedipine for local use in conservative treatment of anal fissures: preliminary results of a multicenter study. *Dis. Colon Rectum,42*,1011–1015.

[43] Shrivastava UK. Jain BK. Kumar P. Saifee Y.A. (2007) comparison of the effects of diltiazem and glyceryl trinitrate ointment in the treatment of chronic anal fissure: a randomized clinical trial. *Surg. Today,37*,482-5.

[44] Ho K.S. Ho Y.H. (2005) Randomized clinical trial comparing oral nifedipine with lateral anal sphincterotomy and tailored sphincterotomy in the treatment of chronic anal fissure. *Br. J. Surg.,92*,403–408.

[45] Agaoglu N. Cengiz S. Arslan M.K. Turkyilmaz S. (2003) Oral nifedipine in the treatment of chronic anal fissure. *Dig. Surg.,20*,452–456.

[46] Ansaloni L. Bernabe A. Ghetti R. Riccardi R. Tranchino R.M. Gardini G. (2002) Oral lacidipine in the treatment of anal fissure. *Tech. Coloproctol.,6*, 79–82.

[47] Prins H.A. Gosselink M.P. Mitales L.E. et al (2005) The effect of oral administration of L-arginine on anal resting pressure and anodermal blood flow in healthy volunteers. *Tech. Coloproctol.,9*,229–232.
[48] Gosselink M.P. Darby M. Zimmerman D.D. Gruss H.J. Schouten W.R. (2005) Treatment of chronic anal fissure by application of L-arginine gel: a phase II study in 15 patients. *Dis. Colon Rectum,48,* 832–837.
[49] Ahmad J. Andrabi S.I. Rathore M.A. (2007) Comparison of topical glyceryl trinitrate with lignocaine ointment for treatment of anal fissure. A randomised controlled trial. *Int. J. Surg.,5,*429-432.
[50] Watson A. Al-Ozairi O. Fraser A. Loudon M. O'Kelly T. (2002) Nicorandil associated anal ulceration. *Lancet,360,*546–547.
[51] Toquero L. Briggs C.D. Bassuini M.M. Rochester J.R. (2006) Anal ulceration associated with nicorandil: case series and review of the literature. *Colorectal. Dis.,8,*717–720.
[52] Pitt J. Dawson P.M. Hallan R.I. Boulos P.B. (2001) A doubleblind randomized placebo-controlled trial of oral indoramin to treat chronic anal fissure. *Colorectal. Dis.,3,*165–168.
[53] Aygen E. Camci C. Durmus A.S. et al (2005) Inhibitory effects of sildenafil citrate on the tonus of isolated dog internal anal sphincter. *Dis. Colon Rectum,48*, 1615–1619.
[54] Torrabadella L. Salgado G. Burns R.W. Berman I.R. (2004) Manometric study of topical sildenafil (Viagra) in patients with chronic anal fissure: sildenafil reduces anal resting tone. *Dis. Colon Rectum,47,* 733–738.
[55] De Godoy M.A. Dunn S. Rattan S. (2004) Evidence for the role of angiotensin II biosynthesis in the rat internal anal sphincter tone. *Gastroenterology,127,*127–138.
[56] De Godoy M.A. Rattan S. (2005) Autocrine regulation of internal anal sphincter tone by renin-angiotensin system: comparison with phasic smooth muscle. *Am. J. Physiol. Gastrointest. Liver Physiol.,289,*G1164–G1175.
[57] Khaikin (2007) Topical captopril cream: a new treatment for anal fissure? The first human study. *Dis. Colon Rectum,50,*747.
[58] Jonas M. Neal K.R. Abercrombie J.F. Scholefield J.H. (2001) A randomized trial of oral vs. topical diltiazem for chronic anal fissures. *Dis. Colon Rectum 44*, 1074-8.

In: Anal Fissure
Editors: P. Sileri and A. L. Gaspari
ISBN: 978-1-61209-716-9
© 2012 Nova Science Publishers, Inc

Chapter 3

BOTULINUM TOXIN AND ANAL FISSURE

Oliver Jones[1]
Oxford Radcliffe NHS Trust, Surgery and Diagnostics,
Churchill Hospital, Old Road, Headington, Oxford, United Kingdom

ABSTRACT

Botulinum toxin is being increasingly used in a wide variety of clinical applications. In anal fissure, its use ranges from first line therapy, for patients failing topical treatments and in combination with surgical approaches such as fissurectomy. It has the advantages of being given as a single treatment overcoming compliance issues that have been seen with topical treatments such as glyceryl trinitrate. It has a good safety profile and few side effects. Perhaps most importantly, its effects at lowering sphincter pressures seem to be limited to about three months. Whilst more data are needed, there appear to be few reports of long term effects of botulinum toxin on continence.

INTRODUCTION

The anaerobic bacillus Clostridium botulinum secretes seven known serotypes of botulinum toxin, typed alphabetically A to G. Its most notorious

---

[1] Oliver Jones DM FRCS: Consultant Colorectal Surgeon, Oxford Radcliffe NHS Trust, Surgery and Diagnostics, Churchill Hospital, Old Road, Headington, Oxford OX3 7LJ. Tel no +441865 235696. E: oliverjones10@hotmail.com.

association is with the disease botulism, which was first described in the early nineteenth century following outbreaks of poisoning from the ingestion of blood sausages. Typically, patients afflicted with botulism suffer with a rapidly progressive paralysis with respiratory failure being a common mode of death.

The earliest clinical application of botulinum toxin was reported in 1980 when it was used for strabismus. [1] Its initial use in the treatment of anorectal disease was reported in an open label study of 12 patients with chronic anal fissure. Each received five units of botulinum toxin into the external anal sphincter. [2] After three months, ten of these patients demonstrated healing. Since then, there has been increasing interest in its applications in colorectal diseases.

MECHANISM OF ACTION OF BOTULINUM TOXIN

On Striated Muscle

The botulinum toxins are 150kd single chain polypeptides that undergo protease mediated nicking to form heavy and light chains. Heavy chains bind irreversibly to the SV2 receptor on the presynaptic membrane enabling the toxin to enter the axon terminal.[3] Once inside the axon terminal, the light chains act to prevent the exocytosis of acetylcholine, through an interference with the SNARE protein complex.[4] The SNARE protein complex allows for the fusion of intra-axonal vesicles with the presynaptic membrane. Thus, botulinum toxin reduces pre-synaptic outflow of acetylcholine at the neuromuscular junction and muscle contraction reduces.

As soon as acetylcholine release from the axon terminal is reduced, the process of recovery begins. This comes about by new nerve sprouting from the nodes of Ranvier in the region preceding the presynaptic membrane. New neuromuscular junctions are formed with adjacent muscle.

In the Context of Anal Fissure

Most of the work on the mechanism of action of botulinum toxin has focused on its effects on striated muscle. However, in anal fissure, the pathophysiological process is spasm of the smooth muscle internal anal sphincter.[5] Anorectal physiology on patients with anal fissure undergoing boulinum toxin injection show there to be a reduction in resting pressure with an insignificant effect on squeeze pressure.[6-8] This is puzzling in that it implies an action of the drug at the site of the internal anal sphincter as this is the predominant determinant of resting pressure.[9] Furthermore, acetylcholine released from the neuromuscular junction of the internal anal sphincter causes a relaxation of the muscle.[10] If botulinum toxin were acting at this level in the internal sphincter, a rise and not a fall in the resting pressure would be expected.

The mechanism of action of botulinum toxin on the internal anal sphincter was studied in the pig both in vivo and in vitro by the Oxford group. In the first of these studies, eight pigs were split into two groups of four each. Four were injected with botulinum toxin into the internal anal sphincter whilst four acted as controls. Between four and six weeks after injection, pigs were slaughtered and the physiology and pharmacology of the internal anal sphincter studied using the superfusion organ bath.[11] The study found that strips from the internal anal sphincter muscle of treated pigs generated significantly less myogenic tone compared to control pigs. Furthermore, the response to field stimulation showed significantly less contraction when parameters were set to activate sympathetic nerves.[12] Human studies have shown that the basal IAS tone is a combination of both intrinsic myogenic tone and tonic adrenergic neural input.[13] Further studies from the Oxford group of porcine internal sphincter strips in vitro have shown again an effect on sympathetic nerve function in the internal anal sphincter with a precise mechanism probably involving a reduction of noradrenaline release at the neuromuscular junction.[14]

DIFFERENT PREPARATIONS OF BOTULINUM TOXIN

There are a number of different commercial preparations of botulinum toxin. The first commercially available preparation was botulinum toxin A, marketed as Botox (Allergan Inc). Subsequently, another botulinum toxin A preparation called Dysport (Ipsen) has been marketed. A preparation of botulinum toxin B is also available, marketed as Myobloc or Neurobloc (Elan Pharmaceuticals). The units of botulinum toxin are derived from the amount required for intraperitoneal injection of a group of mice to kill 50% of the animals (LD_{50}). Despite this, units are not equivalent between different preparations, with, for example, one unit of Botox being equivalent to about 3-5 units of Dysport.[15] This needs to be borne in mind before administration of the drug clinically but also whilst interpreting research studies that use different doses of the various preparations.

EFFICACY OF BOTULINUM TOXIN IN ANAL FISSURE

Efficacy Relative to Placebo

The first randomised trial to compare botulinum toxin with placebo was that of Maria et al. [6] This was a prospective, double-blind, placebo-controlled trial of 30 patients with chronic anal fissure who received either 20 units of botox or saline injection into the IAS. Both groups also received laxatives. After two months, the healing rate in the treatment group was 73%, compared to 13% in the control group, which reached statistical significance. The resting pressure in the treated group was significantly reduced by 25%, whilst that in the placebo group was unaffected. In both groups, voluntary squeeze pressure was unaffected. A further randomised trial comparing botulinum toxin and lidocain pomade also showed a superiority of the botulinum toxin with 71% healing, compared to 21%. [16] However, Siproudhis et al failed to demonstrate any superiority of 100U of dysport at healing anal fissure in their study compared to saline. [17] It is difficult to account for this discrepancy with the Maria et al. paper as dose equivalents were similar, both trials gave laxatives and both trials gave patients injection into the internal anal sphincter either side of the fissure. The result of a meta-analysis [18] of these three trials is shown in figure 1.

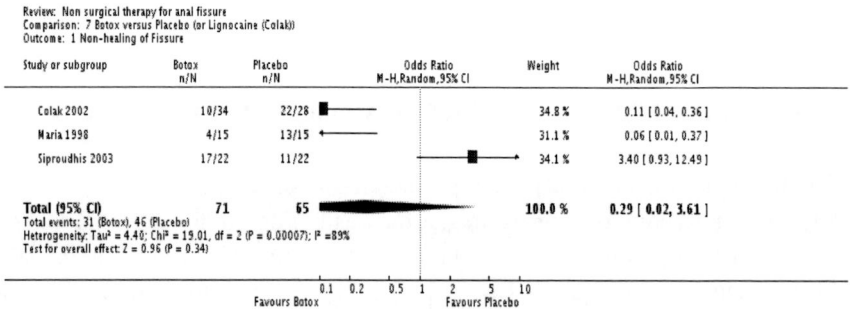

Figure 1. Meta-analysis looking at non-healing of anal fissure in three randomised trials comparing botulinum toxin and placebo (or lignocaine).

Efficacy of Botulinum Toxin as Compared to Sphincterotomy

There have been a number of randomised trials comparing botulinum toxin to sphincterotomy. In the first of these, Mentes et al. [19] randomised patients to receive 20-30U of Botox into the internal sphincter, with the injection repeated at two months if no healing was evident. Patients randomised to the other treatment arm underwent sphincterotomy. 45/61 patients were healed after a single injection of botulinum toxin, with a further eight patients healed after a second injection. Overall healing in the botulinum toxin group was therefore 87% as compared to 98% in the sphincterotomy group, which was not signifncantly different. Eight patients in the sphincterotomy group (but none in the botulinum toxin group) reported anal incontinence. Two further randomised trials have been published by Arroyo et al [20] and Iswariah et al. [21] Both were smaller studies but both showed a significantly lower rate of fissure healing in patients having botulinum toxin as compared to those undergoing sphincterotomy.

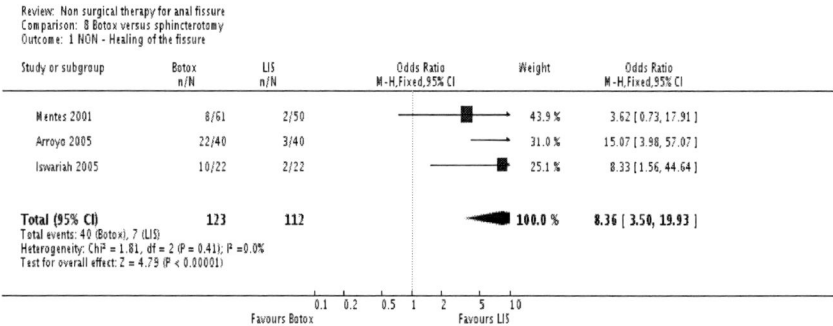

Figure 2. Meta-analysis looking at non-healing of anal fissure in three randomised trials comparing botulinum toxin and lateral sphincterotomy.

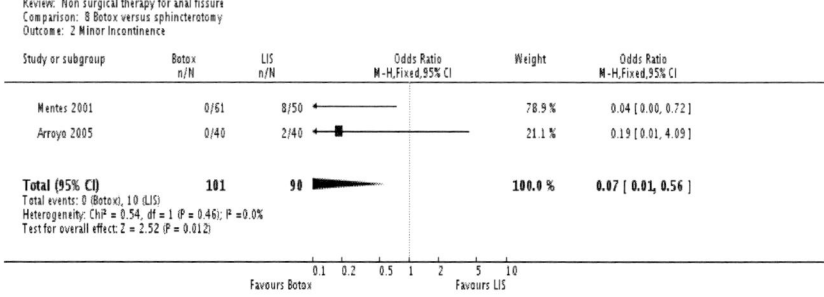

Figure 3. Meta-analysis looking at minor incontinence in two randomised trials comparing botulinum toxin and lateral sphincterotomy.

A recent systematic review of randomized trials comparing botulinum toxin and sphincterotomy for chronic anal fissure examined four studies encompassing 279 patients. It concluded that botulinum toxin was less effective than sphincterotomy in healing anal fissure but that sphincterotomy was more likely to cause minor incontinence. [22] It seems improbable that botulinum toxin will ever be shown to be superior to sphincterotomy, given the effectiveness of the latter technique. However incontinence symptoms in many of the studies looking at sphincterotomy may underestimate the incidence of incontinence. Many symptoms may not been unmasked until many years later, perhaps only as sphincter pressures start to fall with ageing and after the menopause. There is also a Cochrane Review that examines this same issue [18], shown in figure 2 and the risks of minor incontinence with both approaches, shown in figure 3.

Efficacy of Botulinum Toxin Relative to Topical and Oral Treatments for Anal Fissure

The trial of Brisinda *et al* .[23] has suggested that botulinum toxin should now be considered the first line therapy for anal fissure. In this trial, fifty patients were randomised either to 20 units of botulinum toxin into the IAS or 0.2% GTN paste given for six weeks. Healing was found in 96% of patients treated with injection after two months, significantly superior to the 60% healing observed in those using paste. All nine patients who had failed on GTN were retreated with botulinum toxin and all healed, suggesting botulinum toxin, even if not considered first line, may be useful for refractory fissures. Our experience in Oxford of botulinum toxin in "GTN-resistant" fissures has been less favourable, however. In a series of 40 patients treated with 20U of Botox only 43% were healed though a further 30% were rendered asymptomatic without healing. [24]

There have been three other randomised trials comparing botulinum toxin and GTN as primary treatment for anal fissure. [25-27] None showed a statistically significant difference between the treatments and none achieved quite the high rates of healing seen in the Brisinda study. A recent meta-analysis of randomised trials comparing glyceryl trinitrate and botulinum toxin concluded that the two treatments were equivalent in terms of healing but that botulinum toxin had a lower rate of side effects.

Lysy *et al.* [8] have shown a similar result with the topical nitric oxide donor isosorbide dinitrate (ISDN), having shown that in patients with fissures failing to heal with ISDN as first line therapy, second line treatment with botulinum toxin produces good healing rates, and botulinum toxin is even more effective if combined with further ISDN. Similar findings have been reported from another study by Witte and Klaase. [28] The outcome of a Cochrane review [18] examining this issue is shown in figure 4.

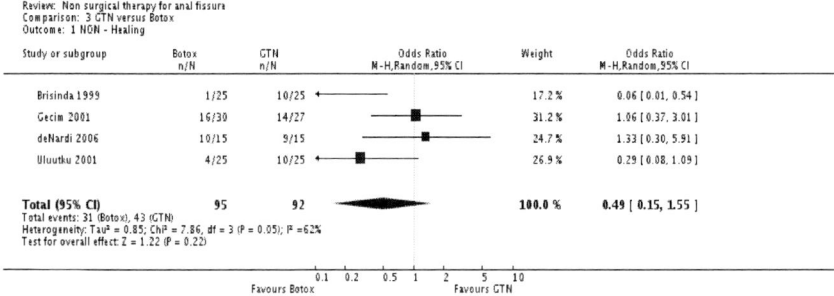

Figure 4. Meta-analysis looking at non-healing of anal fissure in four randomised trials comparing glyceryl trinitrate and botulinum toxin.

The reasons for the apparent superior efficacy of botulinum toxin over GTN are not known. As a single injection, the use of botulinum toxin circumvents any issues of patient compliance. Furthermore, although botulinum toxin's effects last only some three or four months, being reversed by growth of new axon terminals, [29] marked short-term tachyphylaxis is not encountered in the same manner as seen with GTN.

A single randomised trial has compared botulinum toxin and the calcium channel blocker nifedipine (20mg orally for five days). [30] Whilst it showed a trend towards botulinum toxin being more efficacious, this did not quite attain statistical significance.

Relative Efficacy of Different Preparations of Botulinum Toxin

A single randomised trial has compared Botox and Dysport in the treatment of anal fissure. This trial randomised patients to receive either 50U of Botox or 150U of Dysport. It found that healing in the Botox group at two months was seen in 46/50 compared to 47/50 in the Dysport group. No relapses were seen at a mean of 21 months follow-up. The authors concluded that the two regimens were similar both in terms of efficacy and tolerability. [31]

Dose, Site and Method of Injection of Botulinum Toxin

Optimal Dose in Anal Fissure

The optimal dose of botulinum toxin in anal fissure remains controversial. Doses employed range from 2.5 units [32] to 50 units [31]. 20 units of the drug (Botox™, Allergan, High Wycombe, UK) appear to be more effective than 15 units when used for primary therapy of chronic anal fissure, and 25 units is probably superior for re-treatment. [7] Better results were also seen at higher doses (21 units, as compared to 10 or 15 units) in another non-randomised study of chronic anal fissure, in terms of healing rate though this difference did not reach statistical significance. [33] Anecdotally, many centres are giving even higher doses for anal fissure (100U of Botox or 250-500U of Dysport).

Optimal Site for Injection in Anal Fissure

The optimal site of injection of botulinum toxin for anal fissure treatment is another unresolved area of controversy. The external anal sphincter [32], intersphincteric space [33] and IAS [6] have all been used. Whilst there has been no good data supporting one site for injection over another, it does seem reasonable to inject botulinum toxin into the internal anal sphincter as it is spasm of this muscle that is thought to underpin non-healing in most fissures. Certainly, injection into the IAS in the posterior midline appears to be superior to injection in the anterior midline, at least for posterior fissures. [34] Other practitioners inject at the 3 and 9 o'clock positions of the anal sphincter or indeed at the 3, 6, 9 and 12 o'clock positions.

Methods for Injection of Botulinum Toxin

Many clinicians choose to give botulinum toxin injections under general anaesthesia, though the injection is in fact well tolerated in the office setting under local anaesthetic blockade (anal or pudendal nerve block). In patients with internal sphincter spasm, the internal sphincter and the intersphincteric groove are easily identified even without a finger in the anal canal or indeed any other instrumentation. The chosen dose of botulinum toxin can be made up in a small volume of saline (less than 2ml).

A needle-free method of injecting botulinum toxin has been described. This was first examined on fresh porcine specimens before a small open label study was undertaken in ten patients, of whom six of seven who had full follow-up were healed. [35]

SIDE EFFECTS OF BOTULINUM TOXIN INJECTION FOR ANAL FISSURE

Transient incontinence after injection with botulinum toxin has been reported in a number of studies. Its frequency is likely to reflect the patient group and the prevalence of pre-injection symptoms. Furthermore, the more actively the surgeon tries to identify symptoms of incontinence, the higher the likely proportion of patients. Typical symptoms are of flatus incontinence or of urgency. Symptoms are usually short term and tend to occur within the first two weeks of treatment. The rate of incontinence has been reported to be up to 20%. [36] There have been a couple of case reports describing longer term incontinence after injection of botulinum toxin. [37,38]

Rarer complications of botulinum toxin into the anal sphincter have also been reported including Fournier's gangrene in a diabetic elderly man. [39] Antibodies to botulinum toxin A develop in about 10% of patients which has led some to question the safety of repeated injections of the drug. [40] This might be a scenario in which use of botulinum toxin B (myobloc) might be of particular value. There is a single case report documenting a suspected (but not proven) fatal case of anaphylaxis from botulinum toxin given for chronic neck and back pain. [41]

REASONS FOR FAILURE TO HEAL

Not all anal fissures, however, are associated with spasm of the internal anal sphincter. There has been a recent report from Jenkins et al. [42] suggesting that anterior and posterior fissures may have a differing aetiology and pathophysiology. They examined 70 consecutive patients with chronic anal fissure and compared them to 39 asymptomatic controls. They reported that anterior fissures were more commonly seen in young women. Patients with anterior fissures more commonly had a history of obstetric injury and an external sphincter injury demonstrable on endoanal ultrasound. Physiology showed that whilst posterior fissures were associated with a significantly increased maximum resting pressure, resting pressure in those with anterior fissures was not significantly higher. Squeeze pressure was lower in the anterior fissure group. Lindsey et al.[43] have also reported the frequent finding of low pressure fissures. Again, these were commonly found in women and tended to be anteriorly placed. Interestingly, significantly more of the low pressure patients actuallydeveloped no relaxation or even a contractile response to botulinum toxin. There is probably little value in treating the low pressure group with botulinum toxin as presumably the aetiology is not ischaemic.

It is our observation in Oxford that anal fissures resistant to treatment often have an underlying rectoanal intussusception. [44] In this early report, we described 11 patients with average symptom duration of five years, all of whom had failed GTN treatment and additionally either diltiazem, botulinum toxin or both. Two patients had also had a sphincterotomy or manual dilatation. Of these patients, nine complained of obstructed defaecation. On proctography, five patients had recto-anal intussusception. Furthermore, the mean internal sphincter thickness on endoanal ultrasound was 3.5mm, with seven of the patients having a thickened internal sphincter. A thickened internal anal sphincter is highly predictive for high grade internal prolapse.[45]

There is further support for a role of high grade intussusception in resistant anal fissure from a small study of five patients with anal fissure all of whom had failed glyceryl trinitrate or diltiazem and botulinum toxin. They were all subjected to proctography and all five had high grade (recto-anal) intussusception. Three patients also had a rectocoele. All five were healed with a STARR. [46]

FISSURECTOMY COMBINED WITH BOTULINUM TOXIN

It has been reported that the presence of a sentinel pile with an anal fissure is a predictor of poor healing. [47] We had previously noted the same finding in Oxford anecdotally and speculated whether simple injection with botulinum toxin failed to address the chronic fibrosis and scar tissue often seen in association with an anal fissure. We developed the surgical procedure of combining fissurectomy with botulinum toxin. The fissurectomy removed the chronic fibrotic fissure edges and unhealthy granulation tissue in its base, and removed the sentinel pile. This was combined with an injection of 25U of Botox. Our early experience of the procedure described a total of 30 patients who had all failed previous treatments including glyceryl trinitrate and simple botulinum toxin injection. Overall, 93% of patients completely healed with symptoms resolution.[48]

Similar results have been reported from other centres, reporting good healing rates with a low incidence of side effects.[49] There have been reports, however, that relapse rates in the longer term may be as high as 50%. [50] There has been a recent report of healing in all ten patients treated with fissurectomy and botulinum toxin combined with anal advancement flap. [51]

CONCLUSION

Botulinum toxin is a useful adjunct to the many other treatment options available to clinician treating a patients with anal fissure. It is less simple to administer than topical agents and so for many, it is used as second line treatment. Patients failing to heal after botulinum toxin should be re-evaluated and in particular, the presence of other symptoms sought. Where there is a suspicion of Crohn's disease or malignancy, a biopsy should be sought.

The principal issue probably relates to whether or not there appears to be sphincter hypertonia. This may be difficult to assess clinically [52] and anorectal physiology with endoanal ultrasound can be useful in establishing this. Patients with a thickened internal anal sphincter on ultrasound or with significant obstructive defaecation symptoms might benefit from a proctogram. If significant internal prolapse is discovered, this may need surgical correction.

In patients with spasm and significant fibrosis, fissurectomy combined with botulinum toxin may be useful. Those with spasm but minimal fibrosis may simply need a higher dose of botulinum toxin to achieve cure.

Botulinum toxin has few side effects and appears to be well tolerated. More data are needed on its long term safety. Further evidence is also needed on optimal dosage and method of injection. Whilst botulinum toxin is undoubtedly a valuable part of the armamentarium in treating anal fissure, its place relative to other therapies remains controversial.

REFERENCES

[1] Scott AB. Botulinum toxin injection into extraocular muscles as an alternative to strabismus surgery. *Ophthalmology* 1980; 87: 1044-9.

[2] Jost WH, Schimrigk K. Therapy of anal fissure using botulin toxin. *Dis. Colon Rectum* 1994; 37: 1321-4.
[3] Montecucco C, Schiavo G, Rosetto O. The mechanism of action of tetanus and botulinum neurotoxins. *Arch. Toxicol.* 1996; 18:342-54.
[4] Hay JC. SNARE complex structure and function. *Exp. Cell Res.* 2001; 271:10-21.
[5] Brodie BC. Lectures on diseases of the rectum; lecture III; preternatural contraction of the sphincter ani. *London Med. Gazette* 1835; 16:26-31
[6] Maria G, Cassetta E, Gui D, Brisinda G, Bentivoglio AR, Albanese A. A comparison of botulinum toxin and saline for the treatment of chronic anal fissure. *N. Engl. J. Med.* 1998; 338: 217-20.
[7] Maria G, Brsinda G, Bentivoglio AR, Cassetta E, Gui D, Albanese A. Botulinum toxin injections in the internal anal sphincter for the treatment of chronic anal fissure: long term results after two different treatment regimes. *Ann. Surg.* 1998; 228: 664-9.
[8] Lysy J, Israelit-Yatzkan Y, Sestiery-Ittah M, Weksler-Zangen S, Keret D, Goldin E. Topical nitrates potentiate the effects of botulinum toxin in the treatment of patients with refractory anal fissure. *Gut.* 2001; 48: 221-4.
[9] Lestar B, Penninckx F, Kerremans R. The composition of anal basal pressure. An in vivo and in vitro study in man. *Int. J. Colorectal. Dis.* 1989; 4:118-22.
[10] O'Kelly T, Brading A, Mortensen NJ. Nerve mediated relaxation of the human internal anal sphincter: the role of nitric oxide. Gut 1993; 34:689-93.
[11] Brading AF, Sibley GNA. A superfusion apparatus to study field stimulation of smooth muscle from mammalian urinary bladder. *J. Physiol.* 1983; 334:11-2P.
[12] Jones OM, Moore JA, Brading AF, Mortensen NJMcC. Botulinum toxin injection inhibits myogenic tone and sympathetic nerve function in the porcine internal anal sphincter. *Colorectal Dis.* 2003; 5:552-7.
[13] Dickinson VA. Maintenance of anal continence: a review of the pelvic floor physiology. *Gut.* 1978; 19:1163-74.
[14] Jones OM, Brading AF, Mortensen NJ. Mechanism of action of botulinum toxin on the internal anal sphincter. *Br. J. Surg.* 2004; 91:224-8.
[15] Madalinski M. Botox and Dysport are distinct. Endoscopy 2000; 32: 502-3.
[16] Colak T, Ipek T, Kanik A, Aydin S. A randomized trial of botulinum toxin vs. Lidocain pomade for chronic anal fissure. *Acta Gastroenterol. Belg.* 2002; 65:187-90.

[17] Siproudhis L, Sebille V, Pigot F, Hemery P, Juguet F, Bellissant E. Lack of efficacy of botulinum toxin in chronic anal fissure. *Aliment Pharmacol. Ther.* 2003; 18:515-24.
[18] Nelson R. Non-surgical treatment for anal fissure. *Cochrane Database Syst. Rev.* 2006 Oct 18; (4):CD003431.
[19] Mentes BB, Irkorucu O, Akin M, Leventoglu S, Tatlicioglu E. Comparison of botulinum toxin injection and lateral internal sphincterotomy for the treatment of chronic anal fissure. *Dis. Colon Rectum* 2993; 46:232-7.
[20] Arroyo A, Perez F, Serrano P, Lacueva J, Calpena R. Surgical versus chemical (botulinum toxin) sphincterotomy for chronic anal fissure: long-term results of a prospective randomized clinical and manometric study. *Am. J. Surg.* 2005; 189:429-34.
[21] Iswariah H, Stephens J, Reiger N, Rodda D, Hewett P. Randomised prospective controlled trila of lateral internal sphincterotomy versus injections of botulinum toxin for the treatment of idiopathic fissure in ano. *ANZ J. Surg.* 2005; 75:553-5.
[22] Shao WJ, Zhang ZK. Systematic review and meta-analysis of randomzed controlled trials comparing botulinum toxin injection with lateral internal sphincterotomy for chronic anal fissure. *Int. J. Colorectal Dis.* 2009; 24:995-1000.
[23] Brisinda G, Maria G, Bentivoglio AR, Cassetta E, Gui D, Albanese A. A comparison of injections of botulinum toxin and topical nitroglycerin ointment for the treatment of chronic anal fissure. *N. Engl. J. Med.* 1999; 341: 65-9.
[24] Lindsey I, Jones OM, George BD, Cunningham C, Mortensen NJMcC. Botulinum toxin therapy for chronic anal fissure: second-line therapy after failed GTN. *Dis. Colon Rectum* 2003; 46:361-6.
[25] Gecim I. Comparison of glyceryl trinitrate and botulinum toxin A in treatment of chronic anal fissure: a prospective randomised study. *Program Abstracts ASCRS* San Diego 2001.
[26] DeNardi P, Ortolano E, Radaelli G, Staudacher C. Comparison of glyceryl trinitrate and botulinum toxin A for the treatment of chronic anal fissure: long term results. *Dis. Colon Rectum* 2006; 49:427-32.
[27] Uluutku H, Akin ML, Erenglu C, Yildiz M, Ukraya N. Efficacy of nifedipine, glyceryl trinitrate and botulinum toxin in treatment of chronic anal fissure. *Turkish J. Surg.* 2001; 17:343-50.
[28] Witte ME, Klaase JM. Botulinum toxin A injection in ISDN ointment-resistant chronic anal fissures. *Dig. Surg.* 2007; 24:197-201.

[29] Borodic GE, Ferrante RJ, Pearce LB, Alderson K. Pharmacology and histology of the therapeutic applications of botulinum toxin. IN: Jankovic J, Hallett M, eds. *Therapy with botulinum* toxin. New York: Marcel Dekker, 1994: 119-57.
[30] Uluutku H, Akin ML, Erenglu C, Yildiz M, Ukraya N. Efficacy of nifedipine, glyceryl trinitrate and botulinum toxin in treatment of chronic anal fissure. *Turkish J. Surg.* 2001; 17:343-50.
[31] Brisinda G, Albanese A, Cadeddu F, Bentivoglio AR, Mabisombi A, Marniga G, Maria G. Botulinum toxin to treat chronic anal fissure: results of a randomized "Botox vs Dysport" controlled trial. *Aliment Pharmacol. Ther.* 2004; 19:695-701.
[32] Jost WH. One hundred cases of anal fissure treated with botulin toxin: early and long term results. *Dis. Colon Rectum* 1997; 40: 1029-32.
[33] Minguez M, Melo M, Espi A, Garcia-Granero E, Mora F, Lledo S, Benages A. Therapeutic effects of different doses of botulinum toxin in chronic anal fissure. *Dis. Colon Rectum* 1999; 42: 1016-21.
[34] Maria G, Brisinda G, Bentivoglio AR, Cassetta E, Gui D, Albanese A. Influence of botulinum toxin site of injections on healing rate in patients with chronic anal fissure. *Am. J. Surg.* 2000; 179: 46-50.
[35] Bhardwaj R, Drye E, Vaizey C. Novel delivery of botulinum toxin for the treatment of anal fissures. *Colorectal Dis.* 2006; 8:360-4.
[36] Algaithy ZK. Botulinum toxin versus surgical sphincterotomy in females with chronic anal fissure. *Saudi Med. J.* 2008; 29:1260-3.
[37] Brown SR, Matabudul Y, Shorthouse AJ. A second case of long-term incontinence following botulinum toxin injection for anal fissure. *Colorectal Dis.* 2006; 8:452-3.
[38] Smith M, Frizelle F. Long-term faecal incontinence following the use of botulinum toxin. *Colorectal Dis.* 2004; 6:526-7.
[39] Mallo-Gonzalez N, Lpoez-Rodriguez R, Fentes DP, Campos-Franco J, Lado FL, Alende-Sixto MR. Fournier's gangrene following botulinum toxin injection. *Scand. J. Urol. Nephrol.* 2008; 42:301-3.
[40] Hallett M. One man's poison-clinical applications of botulinum toxin. *N. Engl. J. Med.* 1999; 341:118-20.
[41] Li M, Goldberger BA, Hopkins C. Fatal case of BOTOX-related anaphylaxis. *J. Forensic. Sci.* 2005; 50:169-72.
[42] Jenkins JT, Urie A, Molloy RG. Anterior anal fissures are associated with occult sphincter injury and abnormal sphincter function. *Colorectal Dis.* 2007; 10:280-5.

[43] Lindsey I, Jones OM, Cunningham C. A contraction response of the internal anal sphincter to botulinum toxin: does low-pressure chronic anal fissure have a different pathopysiology? *Colorectal Dis.* 2010 (in press).
[44] Wijffels N, Collinson R, Cunningham C, Lindsey I. Rectoanal intussusception frequently underlies recalcitrant chronic anal fissures. *Colorectal Dis.* 2008; 10 (suppl 2):15.
[45] Marshall M, Halligan S, Fotheringham T, Bartram C, Nicholls RJ. Predictive value of internal anal sphincter thickness for diagnosis of rectal intussusception in patients with solitary rectal ulcer syndrome. *Br. J. Surg.* 2002; 89:1281-5.
[46] Clarke AD, Chand M, Tarver D, Nash GF, Lamparelli M. Stapled transanal rectal resection in the management of resistant anal fissures. *Colorectal Dis.* 2008; 10 (suppl 1): 6.
[47] Pitt J, Williams S, Dawson PM. Reasons for failure of glyceryl trinitrate treatment of chronic fissure-in-ano: a multivariate analysis. *Dis. Colon Rectum* 2001; 44:864-7.
[48] Lindsey I, Cunningham C, Jones OM, Francis C, Mortensen NJ. Fissurectomy-botulinum toxin: a novel sphincter sparing procedure for medically resistant chronic anal fissure. *Dis. Colon Rectum* 2004; 47:1947-52.
[49] Scholz T, Hetzer FH, Dindo D, Desmartines N, Clavien PA, Hahnloser D. Long-term follow-up after combined fissurectomy and botox injection for chronic anal fissures. *Int. J. Colorectal Dis.* 2007; 22:1077-81.
[50] Baraza W, Boereboom C, Shorthouse A, Brown S. The long-term efficacy of fissurectomBaraza W, Boereboom C, Shorthouse A, Brown S. The long-term efficacy of fissurectomand botulinum toxin injection for chronic anal fissure in females. *Dis. Colon Rectum* 2008; 51:239-43.
[51] Patti R, Fama F, Tornambe A, Asaro G, Di Vita G. Fissurectomy combined with anoplasty and injection of botulinum toxin in treatment of anterior chronic anal fissure with hypertonia of internal anal sphincter: a pilot study. *Tech. Coloproctol.* 2010; 14:31-6.
[52] Jones OM, Ramalingam T, Lindsey I, Cunningham C, George BD, *Mortensen NJMcC Digital rectal examination.*

In: Anal Fissure ISBN: 978-1-61209-716-9
Editors: P. Sileri and A. L. Gaspari © 2012 Nova Science Publishers, Inc

Chapter 4

CURRENT SURGICAL MANAGEMENT OF ANAL FISSURE

Jason W. Allen and Herand Abcarian
Division of Colon and Rectal Surgery, Department of Surgery,
University of Illinois at Chicago, Chicago, IL, US

ABSTRACT

Fissure-in-ano is a common and distressing disorder for which several surgical procedures have been devised. Operative techniques used to treat anal fissures include: anal stretch, midline internal sphincterotomy, excision of the fissure with or without skin coverage, and "open" or "closed" lateral internal sphincterotomy (LIS). Although some new concerns have been raised about associated post-operative fecal incontinence, LIS remains the gold standard for surgical management of chronic anal fissure.

INTRODUCTION

Fissure-in-ano most likely begins as an acute tear in the anoderm, most commonly from over-distension of the anus from the passage of large or hard stool. The posterior midline segment of the internal sphincter is relatively unprotected and unsupported given the angulation of the anal canal and the elliptical shape of the superficial external sphincter. These particulars correlate well with the typical posterior midline location of anal fissure. The anterior segment of the sphincter in women is unprotected and permits anterior fissures to occur more frequently in this patient population. The healing of midline fissures is hampered by the relative hypoperfusion and ischemia of the anal lining in the midline and is aggravated by sphincter spasm or contracture [1].

As acute anal fissures persist into chronic fissures, the anoderm ulcerates exposing the whitish circular fibers of the internal anal sphincter. The exposed pale tissue of the internal sphincter was historically thought to a fibrotic ring termed the "pecten band" by Miles [2]. Numerous studies have proven beyond doubt that it is the spastic, scarred, and prominent lower edge of the internal anal sphincter that forms the base of the anal fissure [2, 3, 4]. The ensuing ulceration undermines the skin and is secondarily infected which results in the formation of the characteristic sentinel pile and hypertrophied anal papilla of a chronic anal fissure. If this secondary infection continues, it may form a low posterior midline anal abscess and subsequent fistula along with the anal fissure. Once this stage is reached, conservative management is no longer indicated nor successful and surgery is advisable with the primary goal of treating the fistula-in-ano.

SURGICAL PROCEDURES FOR TREATMENT OF ANAL FISSURE

Anal Dilation

Anal stretch was first described as a treatment for fissure-in-ano by Recamier in 1829, who was first to describe this condition. Anal dilation for anal fissure was initially favored by Goligher for treatment of anal fissure and was popularized by Lord for treatment of various anorectal disorders [5, 6]. The technique described by Goligher involved dilation of the anal canal with a bivalve speculum and then dilating the anal canal with two and then finally four fingers for approximately four minutes. In a series of one hundred patients receiving manual dilation, the recurrence rate was as high as 16% and continence defects were seen in 28% of patients. Marby et al published a randomly controlled trial comparing anal dilation versus subcutaneous LIS in 156 patients [7]. Only a little more than half of their patients were seen in four month follow-up, and they report a recurrence rate of 10% and 29% for anal dilation and LIS, respectively. As Nelson indicates in his Cochrane Library systemic review, their follow-up manometry studies revealed increased sphincter pressure in the vast majority patients with recurrent or non-healed fissures that may indicate inadequate sphincterotomy [8]. Inconsistencies in regards to technique, outcomes, and uncontrolled sphincter injuries have caused anal dilation to fall out of favor.

More recently, the use of controlled anal stretch using pneumatic balloon dilation has been investigated by Renzi et al [9]. In a randomized controlled trial of 53 patients comparing balloon dilation versus LIS, they demonstrated a fissure-healing rate of 83.3% and 92% in the pneumatic balloon dilation and LIS groups and incontinence rates of 0% and 16% in the balloon dilation and LIS groups at 24 months, respectively. Although the results of this technique are encouraging, they are yet to be reproduced by others.

Excision of Anal Fissure (Fissurectomy)

Turell considered excision of anal fissure as the "most effective treatment" of an anal fissure. He recommended this procedure for all long-standing and deep fissures and those associated with a skin tag and hypertrophied papillae [10]. In this technique he describes excising the fissure, skin tag, and enlarged papillae together with associated crypt or crypts (Figure 1). The internal sphincter at the base of the wound is then gently dissected to "expose 1.5 to 2 cm of the surface of the sphincter and its fibers are carefully divided at a right angle." With subsequent confirmation of internal sphincter dysfunction as the main cause of anal fissure, it is obvious that the success of fissurectomy is solely related to the midline sphincterotomy rather than the excision of the anal fissure and its associated components.

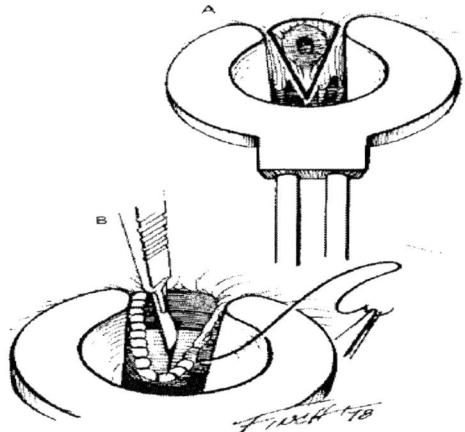

Figure 1. Fissurectomy with partial internal sphincterotomy.

Midline Internal Sphincterotomy

Eisenhammer suggested the division of the internal sphincter for treatment of chronic anal fissure in 1951 [3]. In his paper, he asserts that persistent, chronic spasm of the internal anal sphincter can lead to organic structural changes that gives rise to permanent contracture of the internal sphincter resulting in chronic anal fissures. The area of the fissure is continuously traumatized by defecation and the resultant splitting, healing, and recurrent trauma leads to the chronic anal fissure. In his initial technique, he transected the lower half of the internal sphincter in the posterior midline through the floor of the fissure. Both Morgan and Goligher followed in agreement with Eisenhammer in separate dissertations on surgical anatomy of the anal canal and confirmed the location of the anal fissure on the inferior border of the internal anal sphincter and treated the disorder with sphincterotomy [2, 4]. Midline internal sphincterotomy remained popular until the 1970s.

FISSURECTOMY AND COVERAGE

Gabriel popularized the excision of the fissure-in-ano along with a broad triangular piece of distal anoderm with the apex towards the anus with a division of sphincter in the center of the wound [4]. This wound was left open to heal by secondary intention. Although fissurectomy and posterior midline sphincterotomy have excellent results in relieving pain and low recurrence rates, the healing time for these wounds usually average 7 weeks [11].

Hughes modified Gabriel's operation with the application of a split thickness skin graft to the wound to expedite healing [12]. In his published series of twelve patients, his immediate results showed 100% graft success and wound healing. The major disadvantage of this procedure was the necessity of bowel confinement and hospitalization of the patients for a week. This technique never gained popularity.

Samson and Stewart combined fissurectomy with V-Y advancement flap anoplasty in which a triangular skin flap based outside the anal canal was used to cover the fissurectomy wound (Figure 2) [13]. In their series of 2,072 patients, they report decreased pain and need for wound care compared to standard fissurectomy with a recurrence rate of only 5%. Although this technique decreased the healing time, this procedure had limited popularity in the United States.

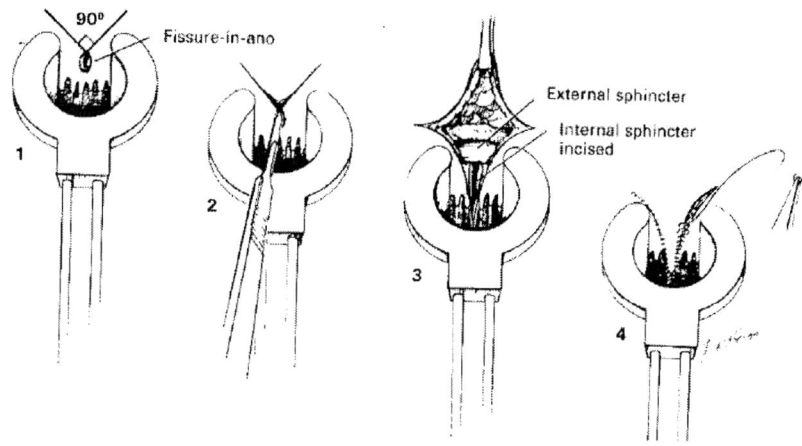

Figure 2. Fissurectomy with V-Y Advancement Flap.

LATERAL INTERNAL SPHINCTEROTOMY

In 1959, Eisenhammer reported a refinement of his technique of sphincterotomy by performing his muscle division laterally or posteriolaterally, because he felt the functional disability was less noticeable than a posterior midline division and the wound healed more rapidly [14]. Bennett and Goligher noted this same effect in 1969 in a report of their series of sphincterotomies for anal fissure in that sphincterotomies performed in the lateral position resulted in minimal functional defects [15]. They also noted in the fecal soilage in 30% of their patients undergoing midline sphincterotomies due to the development of a prominent furrow, or "keyhole deformity", at the site of the sphincterotomy (Figure 3).

In the LIS technique, the patient is placed in the prone "jack-knife" position and, after careful anorectal exam with a bivalve speculum, a linear incision is made from the anorectal verge to the dentate line (Figure 4). The internal anal sphincter is exposed and divided from the level of the dentate line distally. Once hemostasis is obtained, the wound is typically closed with running absorbable suture.

Abcarian reported an initial series of open LIS in 22 patients showing excellent results in patients undergoing LIS [16]. In a later series of 250 patients comparing LIS with fissurectomy plus midline sphincterotomy, the LIS patients fared much better [11]. Hospital stay was shorter (2 days vs. 4 days). Pain relief (1-2 weeks vs. 2-3 weeks) and wound healing (2-3 weeks vs. 6-7 weeks) were faster in the LIS group. The fissurectomy plus midline sphincterotomy patients had an incidence of flatus incontinence in 5% and of fecal soiling in 5% resulting from keyhole deformities. The recurrence rate was 1.5% in both groups with a 1.5% incidence of minor infections in the LIS group.

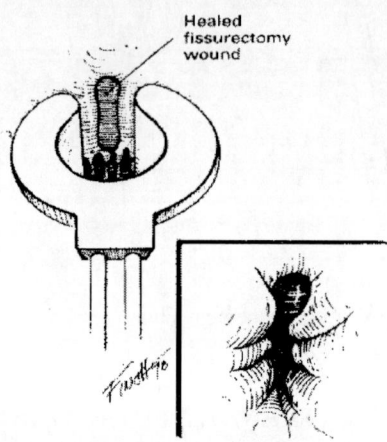

Figure 3. "Keyhole" Deformity.

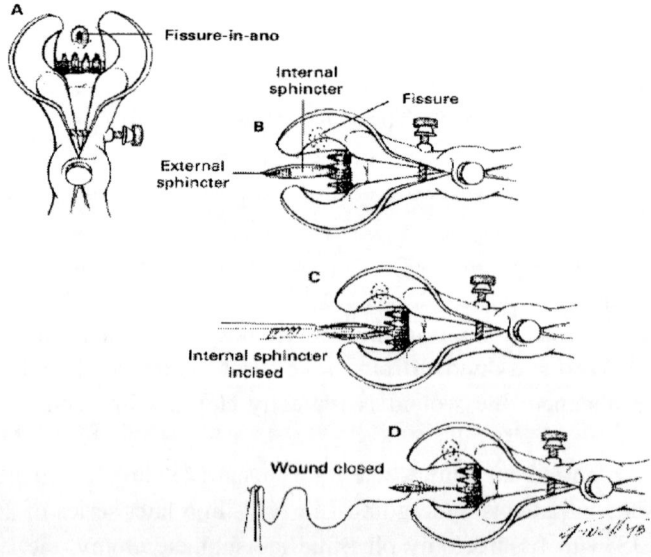

Figure 4. Lateral Internal Sphincterotomy.

SUBCUTANEOUS LATERAL INTERNAL SPHINCTEROTOMY

Subcutaneous lateral internal sphincterotomy avoids a major incision. Parks advocated a lateral internal sphincterotomy through a small circular incision at the anal verge that was sutured closed [17]. To avoid gutter deformities from sphincterotomy, Notares recommended dividing the sphincter subcutaneously in the lateral position using a cataract knife (Figure 5) [18]. In a series of 73 patients, he reported 90% of his patients were pain free in 6 months with fissures healing in 3 weeks in the majority of patients [19]. The incidence of fecal soilage was only 6%.

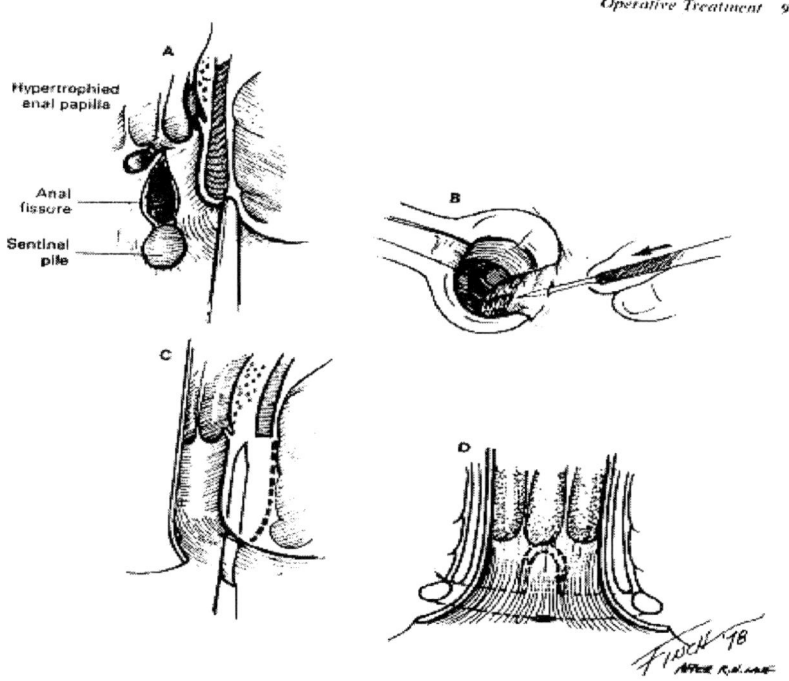

Figure 5. Subcutaneous Lateral Internal Sphincterotomy.

INCONTINENCE CONCERNS

Khubchandani and Reed published a report on their follow-up of LIS patients at their institution in 1989 [20]. Questionnaires were sent to 1355 patients who had undergone LIS in a five-year period from 1980 to 1985. They were able to match surveys and surgical data in 53% of the patients totaling 717 patients. Although the initial healing rate was high (97.7%) and rapid (5-6 weeks) in the patients for which there was surgical data available, the follow-up questionnaires illustrated possible continence concerns. Incontinence of flatus (35.1%), fecal soiling (22%), and fecal incontinence (5.3%) were reported by responders. Although there were several problems with this study including low questionnaire response rate, variable follow-up, no report of patients' pre-operative continence status, and increased incidence of reported complications in the surgical data, this survey illustrated possible problems with post-operative complications with continence after LIS. Garcia-Aguilar et al presented a similar study comparing their long-term results of open versus closed LIS [21]. They also obtained their follow-up data by mailed questionnaires sent to 864 patients who had undergone LIS over a 5 year period. Their overall response rate was 63.5% with both open and closed LIS groups responding at similar rates. Although 90% of their patients reported overall satisfaction with the procedure and a low rate of persistence of symptoms (open group: 3.4%, closed group: 5.3%) and fissure recurrence (open group: 10.9%, closed group: 11.7%), the authors highlight concerns for changes in anal continence in both groups with greater statistical changes in the open LIS group. They report higher rates of loss of control of gas (40.5% vs. 22.8%), soiling of underclothing (30.9% vs. 16.8%), accidental bowel movements (16.7% vs. 3.3%) in the open group when compared with the closed group. Although both surveys suffer from non-respondent bias, these reports helped trigger the investigations into "chemical" sphincterotomies that will be discussed elsewhere in this book.

LATERNAL INTERNAL SPHINCTEROTOMY VERSUS CHEMICAL SPHINCTEROTOMY

A multicenter, randomized, and controlled trial comparing LIS and topical nitroglycerin (NTG) was published by the Canadian Colorectal Surgical Trial Group with excellent results favoring LIS in 2000 [22]. A total of 82 patients were randomized to 0.25% NTG three times daily versus LIS and assessed at 6 weeks and 6 months. Complete healing was achieved in 89.5% of the LIS group versus 29.5% of the NTG group at 6 weeks. Almost 40% of these responders to NTG went on to relapse. At 6 months, 92.1% of the LIS group remained healed compared to 27.2% of the NTG group. The LIS group suffered fewer side effects than the NTG group (28.9% vs. 84%) with one fifth of the NTG group discontinuing the medication secondary to severe headaches or syncope. None of the LIS patients suffered changes in continence.

SPECIAL CONSIDERATIONS

Fissures in Patients with Crohn's Disease

These fissures are usually treated medically because of the fear of postoperative non-healing, worsening infection leading to abscess-fistulas, and anal incontinence. Most patients can tolerate metronidazole at 20mg/Kg in divided doses for treatment. However, at the first sign of paresthesias, metronidazole should be discontinued to prevent permanent neurologic defects. Ciprofloxacin 500mg twice daily may be a good substitute for metronidazole. Recently, "biologics" have replaced antibiotic therapy.

Fissures with Hypotonic Sphincters

Occasionally, an anal fissure is associated with hypotonic rather than hypertonic internal sphincter. If medical therapy fails, fissurectomy without sphincterotomy should be employed to obtain an excisional biopsy. The defect can be left open or covered utilizing V-Y plasty procedure.

CONCLUSION

In the latest permutation of Nelson's Cochrane Library systemic review of the operative procedures for anal fissures, 24 trials including 3475 patients were reviewed [18]. When anal stretch is compared with internal sphincterotomy, anal dilation is associated with a higher risk recurrence and fecal incontinence. Subcutaneous and open LIS procedures show little difference in outcomes for fissure recurrence or incontinence rates when compared. Although much effort is being placed in alternatives to surgical intervention in patients suffering from anal fissures, lateral internal sphincterotomy, because of its efficacy and swiftness of cure, is the gold standard to which all interventions for chronic anal fissure should be compared.

REFERENCES

[1] Schouten WR, Briel JW, Auwerda JJ, et al. Ischaemic nature of anal fissure. *Br. J. Surg* .1996; 83(1): 63-65.

[2] Morgan CN, Thompson HR. Surgical anatomy of the anal canal. *Ann. R. Coll. Surg. Eng.* 1956; 19(2): 88-114.

[3] Eisenhammer S. The surgical correction of chronic anal (sphincteric) contracture. *S. Afr. Med. J.* 1951; 25: 486.

[4] Goligher JC, Leacock AG, Brossy JJ. The surgical anatomy of the anal canal. *Br. J. Surg.* 1955: 43(177): 51-61.

[5] Watts JM, Bennett RC, Goligher JC. Stretching of anal sphincters in treatment of fissure-in-ano. *Br. Med. J.* 1964: 342-343.

[6] Lord, PH. Diverse methods of managing hemorrhoids: dilation. *Dis. Colon Rectum* 1973; 16(3): 180-183.

[7] Marby M, Alexander-Williams J, Buchmann P, et al. A randomized controlled trial to compare anal dilation with lateral subcutaneous sphincterotomy for anal fissure. *Dis. Colon Rectum* 1979; 22(5): 308-311.

[8] Nelson RL. Operative procedures for fissure in ano. *Cochrane Database Syst. Rev.* 2010; (1): CD002199.

[9] Renzi A, Domenico I, Di Sarno G, et al. Clinical, manometric, and ultrasound results of pneumatic balloon dilatation vs. lateral internal sphincterotomy for chronic anal fissure: a prospective, randomized, controlled trial. *Dis. Colon Rectum* 2008; 51(1): 121-127.

[10] Turell R. The surgical treatment of chronic anal fissure. *Surg. Gynecol. Obstet.* 1948; 86(4): 434-8.

[11] Abcarian H. Surgical correction of chronic anal fissure: results of lateral internal sphincterotomy vs. fissurectomy-midline sphincterotomy. *Dis. Colon Rectum* 1980; 23: 31-36.

[12] Hughes, ESR. Anal Fissure. *Br. Med. J.* 1953; 2: 803.

[13] Samson RB, Stewart WRC. Sliding skin grafts in the treatment of anal fissure. *Dis. Colon Rectum* 1970; 13: 372-375.

[14] Eisenhammer S. The evaluation of internal anal sphincterotomy operation with special reference to anal fissure. *Surg. Gynecol. Obstet.* 1959; 109: 583-590.

[15] Bennett RC, Goligher JC. Results of internal sphincterotomy. *Br. J. Med.* 1963: 2(5328): 1500-1503.

[16] Abcarian H. Lateral internal sphincterotomy: a new technique for treatment of chronic fissure-in-ano. *Surg. Clin. N. Am.* 1975; 55: 143.

[17] Parks AG. The management of fissure-in-ano. *Hosp. Med.* 1967; 1: 737.

[18] Notaras MJ. Lateral subcutaneous sphincterotomy for anal fissure- a new technique. *Proc. R. Soc. Med.* 1969; 62: 713.
[19] Notaras MJ. The treatment of anal fissure by lateral subcutaneous internal sphincterotomy: a technique and results. *Br. J. Surg.* 1971; 59: 96.
[20] Khubchandani IT, Reed JF. Sequelae of internal sphincterotomy for chronic fissure-in-ano. *Br. J. Surg.* 1989; 76: 431-434.
[21] Garcia-Aguilar J, Belmonte C, Wong WD, et al. Open vs. closed sphincterotomy for chronic anal fissure: long-term results. *Dis. Colon Rectum* 1996; 39: 440-443.
[22] Richard CS, Gregoire R, Plewes EA, et al. Internal sphincterotomy is superior to topical nitroglycerin in the treatment of chronic anal fissure. *Dis. Colon Rectum* 2000; 43(8): 1048-1055.

In: Anal Fissure
Editors: P. Sileri and A. L. Gaspari

ISBN: 978-1-61209-716-9
© 2012 Nova Science Publishers, Inc

Chapter 5

POSTOPERATIVE COMPLICATIONS AFTER TREATMENT FOR CHRONIC ANAL FISSURE

Giovanni Milito, Federica Cadeddu and Ilaria Ciangola

The Department of Surgery, University Hospital Tor Vergata, Rome, Italy

POSTOPERATIVE COMPLICATIONS AFTER ANAL SPHINCTEROTOMY

Internal sphincterotomy is thought by most surgeons to have minimal complications. Goldberg and co-workers [1] reviewed 306 patients previously submitted to internal sphincterotomy to assess the effective morbidity of internal sphincterotomy. Minor complications were defined as conditions present for more than 1 month and causing symptoms and requiring additional medical consults; major complication were defined as conditions presenting within 3 moths after the operation and requirund reinterventions. Major complications were fistula, bleeding, abscess, or unhealed wounds and occurred in 3 percent of patients. Minor complications were pruritus, persistent wound, pain, bleeding, abscess, discharge, urgency, impaction, or defects of continence and occurred in 36 percent of patients. Long-term follow-up (average 4.3 years) revealed a 22 percent incidence of persistent minor complications. Defects in continence caused 15 percent of total long-term morbidity.

Subsequently, Corman and coworkers [2] in a review of 250 patients submitted to open or closed sphincterotomy recorded a 2.3 percent rate of postoperative infections requiring drainage, one half of which were associated with fistulas. Seventeen percent of patients complained of incontinence for flatus or feces. For two thirds, this was transient.

Faecal Incontinence

Several variations in surgical techniques, i.e., lateral internal sphincterotomy, either open or closed, posterior midline sphincterotomy and anal advancement flap, have been described for the treatment of chronic anal fissure. Lateral internal sphincterotomy (LIS) has been considered, over the last century, the most effective treatment, among the variety of surgical methods described, in order to eliminate internal anal sphincter spasm constantly associated to anal fissure, allowing the ulcer to heal, in over 90% of patients [3]. However, concerns have been raised about either postoperative faecal incontinence and fissure persistence or recurrence, reported in literature in up to 10% of patients [4].

Rate of Incontinence after Internal Sphincterotomy

Some authors have reported high rates of incontinence after LIS. Lewis et al [5] reported some degree of continence in 17% of their patients. Khubchandani and Reed [6] found postoperative soiling in 22% and grade I incontinence in 35.1% of their patients after LIS. Garcia Aguillar and co-workers [7] reported 37.8%, out of 864 patients enrolled, complaining of some impairment of incontinence after LIS. In a large series from Mayo Clinic on 585 patients, Nyam and Pemberton [8] reported some degree of faecal incontinence in 45% of patients at some time in postoperative period. Similarly Casillas [9] reported in a recent study on long term outcomes of lateral internal sphincterotomy in 298 patients, reported temporary incontinence to gas in 31% of patients and persistent incontinence in 30% in absence of impairment of quality of life. In contrast, other smaller series have shown no significant detrimental effects on fecal or flatal incontinence after LIS. Hsu and MacKeigan [10] reported no postoperative soiling or incontinence following lateral sphincterotomy. Actually, the incidence of faecal incontinence reported in literature varies widely from 1.3% to over 30% [3,11]. Moreover, a 1999 meta-analysis including 2727 patients reported similar results of posterior midline and lateral sphincterotomy in terms of fissure persistence or incontinence to faces or flatus [12].

Table 1 Faecal Incontinence After Lateral Internal Sphincterotomy for Chronic Anal Fissure

Authors	Year	N PTS	Incontinence for Flatus (%)	Incontinence for faeces (%)	Incidence of Soiling (%)	Persistence/ Early relapse (%)
Gordon and Vaisilevsky (41)	1985	133	2	1		2
Lewis el al.(2)	1988	350	17	1		6
Khubchandani and Reed (6)	1989	829	35	5	22	2
Melange et al.(42)	1992	76	17	11	9	0
Pernikoff et al.(19)	1994	500	3	1	4	3
Garcia-Aguilar et al.(15)	1996	549	28	8	22	11
Littlejohn and Newstead (23)	1997	287	2		1	2
Hananel and Gorgon (43)	1997	312	1	1	1	1
Nyam and Pemberton (8)	1999	487	6	1	8	4
Argov and Levandosky (44)	2000	2340	2	2		1
Wiley (45)	2004	76	2.7 (at 52 W)	4.1 (at 52 W)	0	5/2,8
Cho (46)	2005	208	10/2	0	0	1/-
Casillas (9)	2005	298	4,4	2,8	0	10,7
Arroyo (4)	2005	40	5(at 1-2-3 y)	0	0	7,5

The wide range of differences seen in the different studies regarding both recurrence and incontinence could be affected by various causes: patients selection criteria, definition of incontinence (it is difficult to quantify and there is no universally acceptable scoring system), follow up length, amount of sphincter sectioned [9].

First of all, the criteria used to define chronic anal fissure are not always the same, so patients with fissures that have been present for a short time with no signs or symptoms of chronicity may be included. In such cases, these patients, in whom healing could be achieved simply by means of conservative hygienic-dietetic measures, are overtreated. According to most authors, chronic anal fissure should be defined as the presence of a fibrous induration or exposed internal sphincter fibers, treated for a minimum of 6 weeks with conservative medical treatment [13].

The amount of sphincter sectioned is also described in various ways in literature [14,15] such as distal half section of the sphincter or 50% to 60% of the muscle, or up to the pectineal line. Therefore, making a comparison between the different surgical results nonsense.

The methods of measuring and collecting data on incontinence are also different among the studies. Questionnaires completed by telephone or sent out by mail reflect rates of incontinence and recurrence that are lower than the true ones, because on clinical examination, asymptomatic patients are frequently found to have persistence of the fissure or certain degrees of mild incontinence that the patient gives no importance. In addition, various incontinence scales are used in the literature that do not reflect both the type (soiling, gas, fluid, solid) and frequency of the leakage. In this respect, the series that do not use a frequency scale and do not include the "soiling," give better results for continence [3,13]. Therefore, Wexner and FISI Scoring System for assessment of fecal incontinence are associated to the most consistent and trustworthy results.

Besides this, after LIS there may be a significant incidence of unreported incontinence related to the shame of patients, who tend to deny some symptoms in the presence of their surgeon and to the mentality of the surgeons who may tend to overlook subtle problems after surgery like seepage or flatus incontinence [7,9].

Finally, follow up time in most prospective studies is shorter than 1 year, so late recurrences and reversible incontinence, the last not rare, are not reflected [9].

Please refer to table I.

Reversibility of Incontinence after Internal Sphincterotomy

Several authors report reversible incontinence in post-sphincterotomy patients.

Nyam and Pemberton [8] described a variation from 45% to 11% after 6 years. Romano and colleagues [16] reported a decrease from 14% to 4.5% after 3 months. In the study of Lewis, in two thirds of patients who experienced postoperative incontinence, this complication was only temporary. Finally, Ram [17] et al reported only 1 patient (2%) with soiling, which resolved after 3 months

The healing process of the anal fissure has been documented also by manometric measurement. McNamara et al [18] demonstrated that resting pressure returns to normal values after sphincterotomy. Ram et al [17], studying the manometric pattern of 50 patients previously submitted to lateral internal sphincterotomy, showed a sharp decline in the anal resting pressure 1 month after the operation followed by a consistent rise in pressure measurements at 3 months follow up. Between 3 and 6 months, there was a marked increase in pressure up to a plateau at 12 months. One year following surgery, the pressure measurements still remained significantly lower than before surgery (but higher than in the controls).

Differently, Arroyo et al [4], studying the manometric pattern 12 months after open and closed sphincterotomy under local anesthesia in 80 patients, reported 5% of the open group and 2.5% of the closed arm with occasional incontinence to gas (p >0.05) and these walues were associated with lower mean resting pressure than in controls (55.1 mmHg vs 80.7 mmHg).

Reasons of Incontinence after Internal Sphincterotomy

Several groups have explored why internal sphincterotomy leads to incontinence in a number of patients. Different factors have been claimed to affect LIS outcomes and morbidities such as previous anorectal surgery, additional procedures, type of surgical technique, length of sphincterotomy, obstetric history among others [9.]

Regarding the surgical technique, the procedure should be controlled and the internal anal sphincter should be divided only partially up to one third, with a consequent limited reduction in mean resting anal pressure of about 25–35 per cent [3,11]. Differently, several ultrasonographic studies have revealed that, like manual dilatation of the anus, internal sphincterotomy appears to be difficult to standardize.

Recently, Sultan evaluated the extent of sphincterotomy with the use of anal ultrasonography [19]. Fifteen patients underwent ultrasonography before and after operation. Nine of ten women and one of five men had inadvertently undergone full-length division of the internal sphincter, and three women complained of incontinence to flatus. Therefore the authors concluded that the length of internal sphincter division in women is frequently greater than anticipated, partly owing to a shorter anal sphincter, and questioned the reproducibility of the procedure.

Subsequently, Lindsey et al [20] noted, using anal ultrasonography, in almost all cases of faecal incontinence following LIS, and over extensive sphincterotomy and sometimes associated to a defect of the external sphincter.

Accordingly, Farouk [21] studied patients complaining of postoperative incontinence after lateral sphincterotomy, evaluated by anal manometry and ultrasonography and noted that sphincterotomy sometimes extends into the external sphincter. Fifteen patients demonstrated an overextensive lateral internal sphincterotomy, of whom eight were women. The sphincterotomy, in 11 cases, was extended to two-thirds of the length, and in four patients the complete length of the internal sphincter had been divided. Only two incontinent patients had a sphincterotomy of 'normal' length; both had an external sphincter injury. In addition, four patients had a sphincterotomy including either internal and external sphincter and seven incontinent women had an underlying obstetric external sphincter injury.

Overzealous or inaccurate sphincterotomy can result in incontinence and women are particularly at risk owing to shorter anal sphincters and occult obstetric sphincter defects that may compound the effects of surgery [3,11,13].

Some chronic fissures are not associated with spasm, making therapeutic reduction in resting pressure not only illogical but also potentially dangerous to continence. Corby [22] examined MRP in women with postpartum chronic fissure and found that median antenatal and postnatal MRPs were 58 and 49 mmHg respectively, similar to those in control patients without anal fissure. The present authors performed manometry on 40 consecutive patients who presented with chronic fissure, and found that 19 per cent of men and 42 per cent of women had low or low-normal resting pressures, placing them at potential risk of incontinence with a surgical reduction in MRP of 25 per cent. It was also noted that surgeons were poor at identifying this at-risk group on clinical grounds.

Tailored Sphincterotomy to Reduce Incontinence Rate

Several surgeons tried to reduce the incontinence risk associated with internal sphincterotomy. Tailored lateral sphincterotomy has been proposed in order to reduce the incontinence risk: the sphincter division is carried cephalad only for the length of the fissure rather than to the dentate with the aim of preserving more sphincter. This procedure appears safe and efficacious, but it has not become common practice. Littlejohn and Newstead [23] reported good results of the tailored lateral sphincterotomy in 287 patients. Flatus, liquid and solid incontinence rates of 1·4, 0·4 and 0 per cent respectively, and a recurrence rate of 1·7 per cent, were observed.

Differently, Ho et al [24] randomly compared lateral sphincterotomy (LAS), tailored sphincterotomy (TS) and nifedipine for the treatment of 132 patients. LAS was significantly more effective than TS in providing pain relief ($P = 0.004$) and better patient satisfaction ($P = 0.020$) at 4 weeks. Surgery (LAS and TS) was associated with significantly better fissure healing rates (both $P < 0.001$ at 16 weeks) and less recurrence (both $P = 0.003$) than nifedipine.

In order to decrease incontinence risk it has also proposed the ultrasound-guided internal sphincterotomy. In an evaluation of ultrasonographically guided internal sphincterotomy, Mylonakis [25] randomized 50 patients to either standard or ultrasonographically guided surgery. There were more complete internal sphincter defects and a greater reduction in MRP with the latter, but healing and incontinence rates were similar in both groups.

Besides this, Pescatori et al [26] fixed the length of sphincter division on the basis of sphincter pattern at anal manometry with minor incidence of continence impairment. Forty patients were randomized to either standard internal sphincterotomy to the dentate line or internal sphincterotomy with the extent of sphincterotomy proportional to the MRP. Postoperative soiling and recurrence were less frequent in the manometry-guided group compared with the standard group (20 and 10 per cent *versus* 5 and 0 per cent respectively). However, benefit from routine anal manometry was not demonstrable in a manometric study conducted before and after operation in 177 patients with chronic fissure.

Clinical Assessment and Diagnostic Testing: Guidelines

Clinical evaluation is crucial to establish a diagnosis and to plan a strategy for the morphofunctional assessment and the treatment of fecal incontinence [27]. All scales for rating severity of fecal incontinence quantify consistency and frequency of stool loss; some scales also incorporate number of pads used, severity of urgency, and the impact of fecal incontinence on quality of life and/or behavioral changes. Nevertheless, none of the several available continence scores has been universally adopted in clinical trials [28,29]. Among others, the Wexner incontinence score, the St Mark's scale and the FISI score are widely used [27].

A complete anorectal examination should be conducted in litothomy position completed by anoscopy and proctoscopy. The positive predictive value of examination for identifying low resting and squeeze pressure is 67% and 81%, respectively [30]. The extent of diagnostic testing is tailored to the patient's age, symptom severity, impact on quality of life and response to conservative medical management.

Anal manometry and endoanal ultrasonography are generally performed. Anal manometry measures resting anal pressure, maximum squeeze pressure and anorectal sensitivity; it assesses the severity of sphincter weakness and the anorectal sensitivity impairment. Ultrasonography documents severity of weakness and identify abnormal sphincter morphology. Pelvic MRI may be also useful; it combines static and dynamic imaging without radiation exposure, is particularly useful for identifying external sphincter atrophy and pelvic organ prolapsed [27].

Keyhole Deformity

Keyhole deformity is defined as mucosal ectropion at the posterior edge of the anus following sphincterotomy. Regarding the incidence, out of 926 patients, Mentes et al [31] described 15 cases of keyhole deformity conservatively treated in 2 cases and surgically treated in 13 cases (9 cases of advancement flap and 4 cases of diamond flap).

Keyhole deformity is proposed to be a historical entity after posterior sphincterotomy. The pathophysiological mechanism underlying the deformity was supposed to be a wide excision of the anoderm, posterior anal skin, and the subjacent muscle fibers [32]. However, current literature revealed cases of key hole deformity following also lateral internal sphincterotomy or conservative treatment for chronic anal fissure. Madalinski and Chodorowski suggested that in this case the lack of vascular relaxing factors and of blood perfusion could alter wound healing and cause the deformity [31].

Clinically patients usually present with the complaints of mucous discharge, pruritus, or soiling that can be misinterpreted as anal incontinence. However, this deformity is not associated with anal incontinence. In rare severe cases, difficult evacuation associated to anal pain, constipation, painful bowel movements, bleeding, and narrow size of the stool and an increasing use of laxatives, enemas, suppositories to manage bowel movements are complained by the patients.

The diagnosis is clinical. If physical examination is painful, exploration under anaesthesia, that may also help to differentiate a functional from an anatomic anal stenosis, is warranted. Adequate examination with anoscopy and proctoscopy may help localize areas of scaring tissue and delineate the feature and extent of the deformity and anal stenosis.

The initial strategy for the management of the keyhole deformity should be conservative, by alteration of the diet, attention to stool consistency, use of enemas after bowel movements, and eventually anal dilatators [31]. Few studies contain limited information about the treatment of keyhole deformity [32]. Surgical repair of the deformities posteriorly, especially in the male, is difficult and, when undertaken, should be done with an appropriate warning to the patient that a good result may not be obtained. Smaller defects are satisfactorily treated with advancement flaps. Bigger deformities should be treated using more complex flap reconstructions, such as diamond flap [33].

COMPLICATIONS AFTER BOTULINUM NEUROTOXIN TREATMENT

Botulinum neurotoxin has been subjected to rigorous clinical evaluation in several randomized, controlled trials and open-label studies across a broad range of therapeutic indications. It is generally well tolerated. After injection, toxin diffuses into the muscles and other tissues. Its effect diminishes with increasing distance from the injection site, but spread to nearby muscles is possible, particularly when high volumes are injected. Distant effects shown by electromyographic tests can also occur, but weakness of distant muscles or generalised weakness, possibly due to Botulinum neurotoxin-A spreading in the blood, is very rare [34].

However, Botulinum neurotoxin-A should be used with caution in patients with disturbed neuromuscular transmission, such as myasthenia gravis or Lambert-Eaton myasthenic syndrome, or during treatment with aminoglycosides. It is contraindicated in pregnancy and while breast feeding. Systemic side effects such as skin and allergic reactions, increased residual urine volume, muscular weakness, abnormalities on electromyography of distant muscles, and postural hypotension have been reported, and BoNT-A diffusion is thought to be responsible for the occurrence of a heart block following treatment for esophageal achalasia in a patient with severe cardiac disease [35]. Other systemic side effects include an influenza-like illness and, rarely, brachial plexopathy, which may be immune mediated. No severe allergic reactions have been reported.

Complications of the treatment have been reported by some authors. Reported side effects, other than mild and transitory incontinence for flatus or feces, encompass perianal thrombosis and hematoma [36]. Some reports have documented detectable abnormalities in some cardiovascular reflexes [37,38].

Table 2. Results of treatment of chronic anal fissure with botulinum neurotoxin

Author/Year	Nr pts	Units/Injection's site	Healing rate (%)	Temporary incontinence (%)	Recurrence (%)	Complications (%)
Minguez et al, 1999[47]	23 27 19	10 B/IAS 15 B/IAS 21 B/IAS	83 78 90	0	37-52	0
Jost and Schrank, 1999[48]	25 25	20 D/EAS 40 D/EAS	76 80	4 12	4 8	0
Brisinda et al, 1999[49]	25 25	20 B/IAS 0.2% GTN	96 60	0	0	0
Fernandez et al, 1999[50]	76	40 B/IAS	67	3	0	1
Madalinski et al, 1999[51]	13	20 B/EAS	-	Nr	15.4	Nr
Khademi and Feldman *, 2000[52]	11	25 B/IAS	82	0	0	0
Maria et al, 2000[53]	25 25	20 B/IAS PI 20 B/IAS AI	80 100	0	0	0
Lysy et al, 2001[54]	15 15	20 B+ID/IAS 20 B/IAS	73 60	0	0	0
Tilney et al, 2001[55]	10	Nr D/IAS		Nr	Nr	20
Jost, 2001[56]	10	200 NB/EAS	0	Nr	Nr	Nr
Brisinda et al, 2003[39]	6	150 D/IAS	100	0	0	0
Mentes et al, 2003[57]	61 50	20-30 B/IAS LIS	86.9 98	0 16	11.4 0	0
Siproudhis et al, 2003[58]	22 22	100 D/IAS Saline	Nr	Nr	Nr	22.7 22.7

*Plus topical nitrates. AI: injection in anterior midline; B: Botox (trade name of the type A preparation manufactured by Allergan, Irvine, CA, USA); D: Dysport (trade name of the type A botulinum toxin preparation manufactured by Ipsen, Maidenhead, UK); EAS: external anal sphincter; GTN: glyceryl trinitrate; IAS: internal anal sphincter; ID: isosorbide dinitrate; LIS: lateral internal sphincterotomy; MVC: maximum voluntary contraction; NB: Neurobloc (trade name of the type B preparation manufactured by Elan Pharma International Ltd, Ireland); Nr: Not reported; PI: injection in posterior midline; RAP: resting anal pressure.

To evaluate safety of this treatment, 6 patients, without detectable cardiovascular or autonomic diseases, who underwent treatment with 150 Dysport units for chronic anal fissure have been studied. Ewing protocol (measurement of heart rate changes during deep breathing, Valsalva maneuver, and during standing up; blood-pressure measurement during handgrip and during standing up) in basal condition (before treatment) and repeated the tests within 96 hours and within 30 days after treatment has been conducted. To classified the severity of the effect on the ANS, a score (0 = normal response; 1 = borderline; 2 = abnormal) is given to each test; an ending score can change from 0/10-1/10 (normal pattern), to 2/10-4/10 (borderline pattern), to 5/10-10/10 (abnormal pattern). No patient had worsening of test scores after BoNT injections. In particular, before treatment a borderline pattern (2/10 score) was found in 4 patients. At 96-hour evaluation, a borderline pattern (2/10 score) was found in 1 patient; at 30 days evaluation, all patients who had previously an abnormal score no longer had such score, and a normal pattern (0/10) was found in all treated patients [39].

Minguez and co-workers [40] analyzed the long-term outcome (42 months) of 57 patients in whom an anal fissure had healed after BoNT injections. The authors state that the late recurrence rate of chronic fissure is high when the BoNT effect disappears. A fissure recurrence has been noted in 22 patients (41.5%). Furthermore, they showed that the highest risk of recurrence is associated with anterior location of the fissure, prolonged illness, the need for reinjection and for high doses to achieve healing.

Please refer to table II.

REFERENCES

[1] Walker WA, Rothenberger DA, Goldberg SM. Morbidity on internal sphincterotomy for anal fissure and stenosis. *Dis. Colon Rectum.* 1985; 28: 832-5

[2] Lewis TH, Corman ML, Prager ED, Robertson WG. Long term results of open and closed sphincterotomy for anal fissure. Dis. Colon Rectum. 1988; 31: 368-71

[3] Utzig MJ Utzig MJ, Kroesen AJ, Buhr HJ: Concepts in pathogenesis and treatment of chronic anal fissure--a review of the literature. *Am. J. Gastroenterol.* 2003, 98: 968-974.

[4] Arroyo A, Perez F, Serrano P, Candela F, Lacueva J, Calpena R. Surgical versus chemical (botulinum toxin) sphincterotomy for chronic anal fissure:

long-term results of a prospective randomized clinical and manometric study. *The American Journal of Surgery* 2005; 189: 429-434.

[5] Nelson R. A systematic review of medical therapy for anal fissure. *Diseases of the Colon and Rectum* 2004; 47: 422-431.

[6] Khubchandani IT, Reed JF. Sequelae of internal sphincterotomy for chronic fissure in ano. *British Journal of Surgery* 1989; 76: 431-434.

[7] Garcia- Aguilar J, Belmonte C, Wong WD, Lowry AC, Madoff RD. Open vs closed sphincterotomy for chronic anal fissure: long-term results. *Diseases of the Colon and Rectum* 1996; 39: 440-3.

[8] Nyam DC, Pemberton JH. Long-term results of lateral internal sphincterotomy for chronic anal fissure with particular reference to incidence of faecal incontinence. *Diseases of the Colon and Rectum* 1999; 42: 1306-1310.

[9] Casillas S, Hull TL, Zutshi M, Trzcinski R, Bast JF, Xu M. Incontinence after lateral internal sphincterotomy: are we underestimating it? *Diseases of the Colon and Rectum* 2005; 48: 1193-1199.

[10] Hsu TC, MacKeigan JM. Surgical treatment of chronic anal fissure. A retrospective study of 1753 cases. Dis. Colon Rectum. 1984; 27: 475-8.

[11] Lindsey I, Jones OM, Cunningham C, Mortensen NJ: Chronic anal fissure. *Br. J. Surg.* 2004, 91: 270-279.

[12] Nelson RL. Meta-analysis of operative techniques for fissure ein-ano. *Dis. Colon Rectum* 1999;42:1424–8.

[13] Madoff RD, Fleshman JW: AGA technical review on the diagnosis and care of patients with anal fissure. *Gastroenterology* 2003, 124: 235-245.

[14] Sultan AH, Kamm MA, Nicholls RJ, Bartram CI. Prospectivestudy of the extent of internal anal sphincter divisionduring lateral sphincterotomy. *Dis. Colon Rectum* 1994; 37: 1031–3.

[15] Garcia-Aguilar J, Belmonte Montes C, Perez JJ, Jensen L, Madoff RD, Wong WD. Incontinence after lateral internal sphincterotomy: anatomic and functional evaluation. *Dis. Colon Rectum* 1998; 41: 423–7.

[16] Romano G, Rotondano G, Santangelo M, et al. A critical appraisal of pathogenesis and morbidity of surgical treatment of chronic anal fissure. *J. Am. Coll. Surg.* 1994;178:600–604.

[17] Ram E, Alper D, Stein GY, Bramnik Z, Dreznik Z. Internal anal sphincter function following lateral internal sphincterotomy for anal fissure. A long-term manometric study. *Annals of Surgery* 2005; 242: 208-211.

[18] McNamara MJ, Percy JP, Fielding IR. A manometric study of anal fissure treated by subcutaneous lateral internal sphincterotomy. *Ann. Surg.* 1990;211:235–238.

[19] Pernikoff BJ, Eisenstat TE, Rubin RJ. Rappraisal of partial lateral internal sphincterotomy. *Diseases of the Colon and Rectum* 1994; 37: 1291-5.
[20] Lindsey I, Jones OM, Smilgin- Humphreys MM, Cunningham C. Patterns of faecal incontinence after anal surgery. *Diseases of the Colon and Rectum* 2004; 47: 1643-1649.
[21] Farouk R, Monson JRT, Duthie GS. Technical failure of lateral sphincterotomy for the treatment of chronic analfissure: a study using anal ultrasonography. *Br. J. Surg.* 1997; 84: 84–85.
[22] Corby H, Donnelly VS, O'Herlihy C, O'Connell PR. Anal canal pressures are low in women with postpartum analfissure. *Br. J. Surg.* 1997; 84: 86–88.
[23] Littlejohn DR, Newstead GL. Tailored lateral sphincterotomy for anal fissure. *Dis. Colon Rectum* 1997; 40:1439–1442.
[24] Ho KS Ho YH Randomized clinical trial comparing oral nifedipine with lateral anal sphincterotomy and tailored sphincterotomy in the treatment of chronic anal fissure.*Br. J. Surg.* 2005; 92: 403-8.
[25] Mylonakis E, Morton DG, Radley S, Keighley MRB. Closedlateral subcutaneous sphincterotomy under directendosonographic control. *Colorectal Dis.* 2001; 3 (Suppl 1): 74.
[26] Pescatori M, Maria G, Anastasio G. 'Spasm-related' internalsphincter in the treatment of anal fissure. A randomised, prospective study. *Coloproctology* 1990; 1: 20–22.
[27] Bharucha AE. Fecal incontinence. Gastroenterology 2003; 124: 1672-1685
[28] Vaizey CJ, Carapeti E, Cahill JA, Kamm MA. Prospective comparison of faecal incontinence grading systems. *Gut.* 1999;44:77–80.
[29] Rockwood TH, Church JM, Fleshman JW. Patient and surgeonranking of the severity of symptoms associated with fecal incontinence: the fecal incontinence severity index. *Dis. Colon Rectum* 1999;42:1525–1532.
[30] Hill J, Corson RJ, Brandon H, Redford J, Faragher EB, Kiff ES. History and examination in the assessment of patients with idiopathic fecal incontinence. *Dis. Colon Rectum* 1994;37:473–477.
[31] Yüksel O, Bostanci H, Leventoğlu S, Şahin TT and Menteş BB. Keyhole Deformity: A Case Series. *Journal of Gastrointestinal Surgery* 2008; 6:1110-1114.
[32] Mazier WP. Keyhole deformity. Fact and fiction. *Dis. Colon Rectum* 1985;28:8–10.
[33] Abcarian H. Surgical correction of chronic anal fissure: results of lateral internal sphincterotomy vs. fissurectomy-midline sphincterotomy. *Dis. Colon Rectum* 1980;23:31–36.

[34] Brisinda G, Cadeddu F, Brandara F, Brisinda D, Maria G. Treating chronic anal fissure with botulinum neurotoxin. Nature. Clinical Practice. *Gastroenterology and Hepatology* 2004; 1: 82-89.
[35] Malnick SD, Metchnik L, Somin M, Bergman N, Attali M: Fatal heart block following treatment with botulinum toxin for achalasia. *Am. J. Gastroenterol.* 2000, 95: 3333-3334.
[36] Lock G, Holstege A. Botulinum toxin in treatment of chronic anal fissure. *Z. Gastroenterol.* 1999, 37: 253-255.
[37] Girlanda P, Vita G, Nicolosi C, Milone S, Messina C: Botulinum toxin therapy: distant effects on neuromuscular transmission and autonomic nervous system. *J. Neurol. Neurosurg. Psychiatry* 1992, 55: 844-845.
[38] Tonkin AL, Frewin DB: Drugs, chemical, and toxins that alter autonomic function. In Autonomic Failure. *A textbook of clinical disorders of the autonomic nervous system.* Edited by Mathias CJ, Bannister R. New York: Oxford University Press, Inc; 1999:527-533.
[39] Brisinda D, Maria G, Fenici R, Civello IM, Brisinda G: Safety of botulinum neurotoxin treatment in patients with chronic anal fissure. *Dis. Colon Rectum* 2003, 46: 419-420.
[40] Minguez M, Herreros B, Espi A, Garcia-Granero E, Sanchiz V, Mora F et al. Long-term follow-up (42 months) of chronic anal fissure after healing with botulinum toxin. *Gastroenterology* 2002; 123(1):112-117.
[41] Gordon PH, Vasilevsky CA. Symposium on outpatient anorectal procedures. Lateral internal sphincterotomy: Rationale, technique and anesthesia. *Can. J. Surg.* 1985;28:228–30.
[42] Melange 1992 Melange M, Colin JF, Van Wymersch T, et al. Anal fissure: Correlation between symptoms and manometry before andafter surgery. *Int. J. Colorectal. Dis.* 1992;7:108–11.
[43] Hananel N, Gordon PH. Lateral internal sphincterotomy for fissure –in-ano revisited. *Dis. Colon Rectum* 1997; 40: 597-602.
[44] Argov S, Levandovsky O. Open lateral sphincterotomy is still the best treatment for chronic anal fissure. *American Journal of Surgery* 2000; 179: 201-2.
[45] Wiley M, Day P, Rieger N, Stephens J, Moore J. Open versus closed lateral internal sphincterotomy for idiopathic fissure-in-ano: a prospective randomized, controlled trial. *Diseases of the Colon and Rectum* 2004; 47: 847-852.
[46] Cho DY. Controlled lateral sphincterotomy for chronic anal fissure. *Diseases of the Colon and Rectum* 2005; 48: 1037-1041.

[47] Minguez M, Melo F, Espi A, Garcia-Granero E, Mora F, Liedo S, Benages A. Therapeutic effects of different doses of botulinum toxin in chronic anal fissure. *Dis.Colon Rectum* 1999; 42: 1016-1021.

[48] Jost, W.H.; Schrank, B. Repeat botulinum toxin injections in anal fissure: in patients with relapse and after insufficient effect of first treatment. *Dig. Dis. Sci.* 1999; 44:1588-9.

[49] Brisinda G, Maria G, Bentivoglio AR, Cassetta E, Gui D, Albanese A: A comparison of injections of botulinum toxin and topical nitroglycerin ointment for the treatment of chronic anal fissure. *N. Engl. J. Med.* 1999; 341: 65-69.

[50] Fernandez, L. F.; Conde, F. R.; Rios, R. A.; Garcia, I. J.; Cainzos, F. M.; Potel, L. J. *Botulinum Toxin for the Treatment of Anal Fissure Dig.Surg.* 1999; 16: 515-518.

[51] Madalinski, M.; Jagiello, K.; Labon, M.; Adrich, Z.; Kryszewski, A. Botulinum toxin injection into only one point in the external anal sphincter: a modification of the treatment for chronic anal fissure. *Endoscopy* 1999; 31: S63.

[52] Khademi, A.; Feldman, D. M. A comparison of combination of botox (botulinum toxin) and nitroglycerin in the treatment of chronic anal fissures *Am. J. Gastroenterol.* 2000; 95: 2538.

[53] Maria G, Brisinda G, Bentivoglio AR, Cassetta E, Gui D, Albanese A. Influence of botulinum toxin site of injections on healing rate in patients with chronic anal fissure. *Am. J. Surg.* 2000; 179: 46-50.

[54] Lysy J, Israelit-Yatzkan Y, Sestiery-Ittah M, Weksler-Zangen S, Keret D, Goldin E. Topical nitrates potentiate the effect of botulinum toxin in the treatment of patients with refractory anal fissure. *Gut.* 2001; 48: 221-224.

[55] Tilney HS, Heriot AG, Cripps, NP. Complication of botulinum toxin injections for anal fissure. *Dis.Colon Rectum* 2001; 44: 1721-1724.

[56] Jost WH. Botulinum toxin type B in the treatment of anal fissures: first preliminary results. *Dis. Colon Rectum.* 2001; 44:1721-2.

[57] Mentes BB, Irkorucu O, Akin M, Leventoglu S, Tatlicioglu E. Comparison of botulinum toxin injection and lateral internal sphincterotomy for the treatment of chronic anal fissure. *Dis.Colon Rectum* 2003; 46: 232-237.

[58] Siproudhis L, Sebille V, Pigot F, Hemery P, Juguet F, Bellissant E. Lack of efficacy of botulinum toxin in chronic anal fissure. *Aliment. Pharmacol. Ther.* 2003; 18: 515-524.

In: Anal Fissure
Editors: P. Sileri and A. L. Gaspari
ISBN: 978-1-61209-716-9
© 2012 Nova Science Publishers, Inc

Chapter 6

ANAL FISSURE: TREATMENT OPTIONS IN PARTICULAR CASES

Stefano D'Ugo, Sara Di Carl, Lodovico Patrizi and Vito Maria Stolfi
Department of Surgery, Tor Vergata University, Rome, Italy

ABSTRACT

Particular anal fissures, multiple or "off the midline", must be viewed with suspicion for underlying pathologies, such as Crohn's disease and HIV/AIDS. Their treatment require specific knowledge, as fissures in women during pregnancy and postpartum.

Fissures associated with Crohn's disease constitute 21-35% of perianal lesions; they can be locally aggressive, progressing to form deep ulcers with granulating bases and overhanging skin edges. The distinctive features are lack of pain and chronicity.

Anorectal disease in HIV patients is the most common reason for surgical intervention. The cause of these conditions is still unclear, and there is no definite consensus on how they should be treated. Fissures are typically painful and usually located in the posterior midline. Wound healing is a major problem after surgery, and $CD4^+$ T-lymphocyte count seems to be a significant prognostic factor regarding this aspect.

Women during pregnancy and postpartum period frequently experience anal fissures, with an incidence of about 9-10%. The majority of them appear during the postpartum period. The most important risk factor identified is dyschezia.

The first line of treatment in these particular cases should be medical management. Surgical intervention should be reserved for those patients who fail to respond to conservative measures.

INTRODUCTION

It is well known that anal fissure is a common proctological problem, about 10-15% of all medical evaluations for anorectal disorders [1]. It occurs most commonly in young adults and affects both genders equally.

This condition may be frequently misdiagnosed as hemorrhoids by primary care providers. Because the symptoms are so typical, its presence can be often inferred from the patient's history alone. Diagnosis is generally established by simple physical examination and does not require anal instrumentation.

The great majority, about 80 percent, is located in the posterior midline [2], although anterior midline fissures are seen in 25% of affected women and 8% of affected men [3]. Those located anteriorly and posteriorly at the same time (3%) or localized in other anal position are rare [4].

The typical anal fissure is often not associated to other colorectal or systemic diseases, and therefore is defined idiopathic; atypical fissures may be multiple or "off the midline", or be large and/or irregular. They must be viewed with suspicion for underlying pathologies such as Crohn's disease, HIV/AIDS, tuberculosis, syphilis, or anal carcinoma.

In this chapter the treatment options are analyzed in such particular conditions, like Crohn's disease and HIV/AIDS; a strategy of management of anal fissure will also be given during pregnancy and postpartum period.

ANAL FISSURE IN CROHN'S DISEASE

The incidence of perianal involvement in patients with Crohn's disease varies greatly, being found from 14% to 38% of patients [5]. In most cases, bowel involvement precedes perianal disease, but as many as four in ten patients can experience symptoms before intestinal involvement manifests [6].

The presence of perianal pathology is associated with a more disabling natural history, with increased extraintestinal manifestations and greater steroid resistance [7,8].

Unlike typical fissures, those associated with Crohn's disease can also be locally aggressive, progressing to form deep ulcers with granulating bases and overhanging skin edges.

Sweeney et al. found that a fissure was most commonly located posteriorly (41%), whereas multiple and lateral fissures occurred in 32-33 % and 9-20 % of patients respectively [9,10].

The prevalence of perianal manifestations increases as the disease progresses distally. This was illustrated by Sangwan et al. who found that the time elapsed between intestinal disease and proctological pathology was shorter for colonic disease and longer for ileal involvement [11]. Perianal Crohn's disease is often recurrent, with 35% to 59% of patients relapsing within 2 years [12]. There is not a predilection for age, since between 13% and 62% of children and adolescents with Crohn's disease will experience perianal manifestations [13,14]; however, a younger age of onset increases the odds of developing perianal disease over time [15].

Proctological pathology, in the absence of rectal inflammation, has a better outcome than disease associated with involvement of the rectum [16]. More than 80% of patients require surgery, and as many as 20% will require proctectomy [5].

Abscess and fistula are the most common presentations of anorectal Crohn's disease (29.5% and 26.7% respectively) [17]. Fissures constitute 21-35% of perianal lesions [11].

In the general population anal fissures usually are symptomatic; however some authors described the distinctive features of all types of perianal Crohn's disease as lack of pain, chronicity, induration, multiplicity, and cyanotic coloration. Moreover the pain frequently, but non always, implies that an abscess is present, and consequently an accurate anorectal assessment is necessary to exclude this condition before starting any treatment [18]. Abcarian et al. described that anal fissures without pain do not require fissurectomy or internal sphincter-otomy [19].

In contrast to manometric findings in patients without inflammatory bowel disease, some authors reported that there is no increase in resting anal sphincter pressure [20].

Platell et al. noted symptomatic anal pathology in 42.4% of Crohn's disease patients; 27.6% of this patients had anal fissure [21]. Sangwan et al. reported that 3.8% of Crohn's disease patients required surgery for symptomatic perianal disease, and 31.8% of these patients had anal fissure [11].

The standard algorithm for anal fissure therapy has traditionally consisted of trial of fiber supplementation, sitz bath and topical analgesics; if the pain is intolerable or if conservative care fails, surgery is performed (usually a lateral internal sphinterotomy). This approach has been modified in the recent years, as a better understanding of fissure pathophysiology has provided a number of novel therapeutic options, like pharmacological sphincter relaxants (topical nitrates, calcium channel blockers, muscarinic agonists, adrenergic agonists and antagonists, botulin toxin).

These fissures are challenging to treat. The first line of treatment should be medical management (including nitroglycerin paste, calcium channel blockers and botulinum toxin); these treatments are successful in up to 80% of cases [22].

Although steroids are commonly used in the treatment of Crohn's disease, there is less evidence to suggest a benefit in perianal disease [23].

Anorectal surgery is thought to be hazardous in this inflammatory bowel disease. Surgeons have traditionally approached the anal canal with caution in Crohn's disease patients, fearing that an operation might precipitate complications leading to proctectomy. Furthermore, therapies requiring sphincter muscle division are perceived as putting the patients at risk for incontinence, as these patients frequently have an underlying diarrhea state and are at significant risk for requiring additional anal surgery in the future. Despite these concerns, the degree of continence impairment after sphincterotomy for fissure has not been systematically studied in patients with Crohn's disease.

Most authorities advocate standard conservative treatment combined with medical or surgical therapy directed at controlling diarrhea as first line treatment for Crohn's fissure. Conservative care leads to fissure healing in about half of all cases. If it fails and the fissure remains symptomatic, the patients should be examined under anesthesia and a sphincterotomy or gentle dilatation should be performed. However, in the presence of proctitis, surgery should be avoided.

To date in the literature there is a lack of randomized controlled trials or guidelines on specific treatment modality of anal fissure in Crohn's patients. Local anorectal procedures used in the management of this condition in the general population, such as dilatation of the sphincter or sphincterotomy, have been reported infrequently in Crohn's disease, also because of poor wound healing in these patients.

Wolkomir and Luchtefeld in a study of 25 patients who had Crohn's disease with symptomatic fissure, reported that 22 had completely healed by 2 months following sphincterotomy. No patients had a direct complication from operative therapy and only 3 eventually required proctectomy for severe recurrent disease [24].

Fleshner et al. reviewed a series of 56 patients with Crohn's disease and anal fissure; 49% healed after medical therapy, 88% after anorectal surgery, and 29%

after abdominal surgery. In addition, 25% of patients who had unhealed fissures that did not undergo lateral internal sphincterotomy went on to develop an abscess or fistula from the base of the fissure, leading the authors to propose a more liberal use of LIS for fissure not responding to medical therapy. However, results with respect to continence were not reported [10].

Despite these reports, given the continence risks associated with surgery, medical management is the preferred initial therapy in patients who have Crohn's related fissures. Surgical intervention should be reserved for those patients who have minimal active anorectal inflammation, after failure of conservative therapy. During the surgical procedure, division of sphincter muscle should be kept to a minimum [22].

Limited numbers of patients who undergone anal dilatation for Crohn's fissure have been reported. Sweeney et al. reported good results with dilatation of the sphincter in two patients with Crohn's disease and anal fissure [9]. Allan et al. described 7 of such patients; 4 improved and 1 was rendered incontinent [25]. Fleshner et al. in their study of 56 patients, 49 with symptomatic fissures, believed that dilatation of the sphincter should be avoided in Crohn's disease, not only because of suboptimal healing of the fissure, but also to avoid uncontrolled trauma to diseased anal mucosa with the potential for development of secondary infection of fistula [10].

Although in the literature there are few data on this argument, it seems that many anal fissures in patients with Crohn's disease will heal using medical measures only; however local anorectal operations are safe in carefully selected patients with refractory anal fissure disease. The surgical procedure should create small wounds and minimize the damage to the diseased mucosa and external sphincter. Closed subcutaneous lateral internal sphincterotomy is ideally suited for this purpose. Fissurectomy may be considered only when the edges of the fissure are densely fibrotic and are unlikely to heal after sphincterotomy alone.

ANAL FISSURE IN HIV/AIDS PATIENTS

Human immunodeficiency virus (HIV) infection is pandemic in both the United States and the world. Infection rates have levelled off in many populations in which rates have been historically high, but other societies previously unaffected by the disease are seeing dramatic increases. This is especially true among heterosexuals.

Anorectal disease affects 5.9% to 34% of homosexual males infected with the HIV; this incidence is much higher than in the general community [26,27]. It's the most common reason for surgical intervention in these individuals [28], being estimated that more than one-half of these patients will require surgical treatment for their anorectal condition [17].

In homosexual HIV positive patients trauma secondary to anoreceptive intercourse and/or HIV associated diarrheal states predisposes to fissures.

Several studies have examined the clinical course of anorectal disease in patients infected with HIV, but the cause of these conditions is still unclear, and there is no definite consensus on how they should be treated.

Early studies about HIV infected patients with perianal disease noted poor healing and high morbidity rates than seronegative people. Recent changes in the systemic treatment of HIV infection and newer drug regimens that include combinations of protease inhibitors and nucleoside analogs have greatly improved the prognosis for HIV infected patients [29]. The outcome of surgical treatment of perianal disorders might ameliorate in the setting of these new drug regimens [30,31]. Moreover, earlier HIV diagnosis, greater physician awareness, prophylaxis and better overall patient compliance and education have a role in this advancement.

Little specific literature is available on HIV associated fissures, and detailed reports of function after surgery are nonexistent. In addition, no data have been reported regarding use of topical sphincter relaxants or botulin toxin in HIV positive patients.

The results of wound healing after operation have varied considerably, from less than half of all patients infected with HIV healing their wounds within 6 months, often because of death of the patient, to 94% healing in other experiences [28, 32].

Ulcerative processes of the anorectum in HIV positive patients are common and extremely debilitating. The spectrum runs from "benign" anal fissures to AIDS-specific "idiopathic" anal ulcers, and these entities must be differentiated from each other, since they share certain features. Either are typically painful; fissures are associated with pain on defecation, whereas idiopathic ulcers produce a more persistent and "gnawing" pain. Both processes are usually in the posterior midline of the anal canal.

However, fissures in seropositive people are usual indistinguishable from those in the seronegative population, which are distal in the anal canal, frequently associated with sentinel tags, narrow, shallow, not invasive, and associated with a hypertonic anal sphincter. In contrast, idiopathic anal ulcers tend to be more proximal in the anal canal, associated with a patulous anus (due to sphincteric destruction), broad-based with occasional mucosa bridging, and deeply invasive.

Management of HIV infected patients with perianal disorders is challenging.

Surgeons are faced with a dilemma. They must decide between a conservative approach, based on fears of perioperative morbidity, or an aggressive approach, based on concerns of severe septic complications resulting from untreated disease.

Nowadays, aggressive surgical intervention of HIV associated to anorectal disorders should be individualized to obtain the best result. Fissures coincident with HIV can be safely and effectively treated with standard methods used in the seronegative population.

Viamonte et al. reported their results of 219 HIV positive patients with diagnosis of anorectal pathology; thirty-three of them were identified as having benign fissures. All were treated as if HIV negative, with conservative medical therapy initially and later internal sphincterotomy after failure of medical therapy. Ten patients improved on conservative therapy; ten were lost to follow-up. Of 13 patients who underwent LIS after two to six weeks of failure of conservative measures, 12 improved. There were no post-operative infections or incontinence [33].

Wound healing is a significant problem after anorectal operations in patients infected with HIV. Different studies correlated $CD4^+$ T-lymphocyte count and CD4/CD8 ratios to wound healing after surgery, however without a certain predictive value.

Consten et al. analyzed 83 HIV positive patients with anorectal pathology and reported a correlation between low preoperative CD4 count and disturbed wound healing [34].

Lord R. analyzed the factors associated with delayed wound healing in one hundred one patients infected with HIV undergone to 161 anorectal operations. Anal fissures were found in thirty-eight patients; thirty of these were chronic fissures, with deep, wide fissuring and, in some cases, a sentinel pile and skin tag. Only eight patients presented typical acute anal fissure. Chronic lesions were situated most commonly in the midline, especially the posterior position. Lateral internal sphincterotomy, anal dilatation, or both of them were performed.

This study confirms that the wound healing is a significant problem after anorectal surgery because only a minority of wounds were healed three months after operation; in this series only 16% of patients had healed at the end of follow-up.

Both patients with and without AIDS manifested delayed wound healing, and stage of HIV illness was not a significant predictor of wound healing. Particularly the length of time between HIV diagnosis and first operation was not significant, but wound healing was significantly better in patients who had been diagnosed with AIDS more than 1 year before operation, compared with those operated on within the first year after diagnosis of AIDS.

Why the interval AIDS diagnosis and date of operation influences wound healing is not clear.

The CD4 count was a significant prognostic factor for wound healing. Patients with $CD4^+$ T-lymphocyte counts < 50/µL were more than four times more likely to have unhealed wounds at three months compared with when the CD4 count was above 50/µL.

Impaired wound healing in patients with low numbers of $CD4^+$ T-lymphocytes may be related to the failure of infected or depleted T cells to produce cytokines important in normal wound healing.

Patients with chronic fissures had a significantly lower median CD4 count than other HIV subjects, and their rate of wound healing was lowest of all anorectal lesions [32].

To treat anal fissure in HIV/AIDS patients several operative methods were used, mainly LIS and anal dilatation, but none seems to have been really effective.

ANAL FISSURE DURING PREGNANCY AND POSTPARTUM PERIOD

Anal fissures are common and are responsible for severe discomfort during pregnancy and puerperium. To date, scientific epidemiologic data are lacking, but fissures are thought to be the second most common anorectal complication of pregnancy after thrombosed external hemorrhoids.

Data analyzed in the literature show an incidence of anal fissure about 9-10% during this period, although some series reported different percentages [35,36].

The diagnosis is suggested by history alone, and visual inspection of the anal margin often confirms the diagnostic hypothesis, demonstrating the classical triad of sentinel skin tag, anal canal ulcer, and hypertrophic anal papilla; however in the acute setting, only the anal canal ulcer is seen.

Unlike fissures in Crohn's disease and HIV/AIDS patients, those during pregnancy are generally located in an anteriorly or posteriorly typical midline position. Nevertheless, there is a slight predominance of anterior localization [37].

The mechanisms underlying this injury are unclear; decreased blood flow in anal mucosa and traumatic events have been suggested to be involved.

Abramowitz et al. analyzed in a prospective study 165 consecutive pregnant females during the last 3 months of pregnancy and after delivery (within 2 months). They reported that the majority of anal fissures appeared during the postpartum period; actually the study showed two cases (1.2%) during the last months of childbearing, and twenty-five (15.2%) after labour. Therefore fissure seems to be rare during the first one and more frequent during the second one period. After delivery, anal fissures occurred homogeneously, with no peak in frequency.

The higher prevalence reported in this study compared to literature data, may have been caused by the longer period of follow-up. Indeed, eight patients developed anal fissure during the last two weeks of follow-up; without these last cases, the incidence would have been 10.3 percent (17/165) [36].

Several reports in the literature demonstrate the importance of some specific condition associated to higher risk to develop anal fissure, particularly traumatic events.

The most important risk factor identified is dyschezia; this condition, also defined terminal constipation, is a difficulty in completing rectal evacuation. It is very common during pregnancy [38,39], but epidemiologic data are lacking.

Corby et al. in their prospective study of 313 primigravid women found that postpartum constipation was the only variable associated with anal fissure after labour. This condition was more common in women who developed fissure (62%) than in those who did not (29%), and this difference was statistically significant ($P < 0.01$). Accordingly they stated that dyschezia was the primary cause and not a secondary effect of acute postpartum anal fissure [35].

Similarly Abramowitz et al. identified terminal constipation the most important independent risk factor for anal fissure. They found that 23 percent of patients (38 pts) had dyschezia during the last three months of pregnancy and 33.3 percent (55 pts) during the postpartum period. Constipation increased by 5.7 the relative risk of anal lesions during this period. Indeed of the fifty-five patients with dyschezia, 21 (38.2%) had anal fissure; conversely of the 110 patients without terminal constipation, only four (3.6%) had the lesion.

Another independent risk factor for anal fissure during postpartum was late delivery. The cutoff point to define early and late delivery was the median duration of pregnancy (39.7 weeks). Late delivery was reported to have an odds ratio of 1.4; therefore patients who delivered after 39.7 weeks of pregnancy were more likely to have anal fissure than those who delivered before that time. The reason for this link was unclear. Delayed changes in the perineum and the duration of hormonal change may predispose females to these lesions [36].

Traumatic delivery also appears to be associated with anal fissure, but in the literature conflicting results have been obtained. In an old study Martin found that primiparous females, forceps deliveries and perineal damage were associated with fissures in the postpartum period [40].

However other reports stated that obstetric factors and mode of delivery did not alter the incidence of fissure and, in particular, the incidence of perineal laceration did not differ between women who did and those who did not develop a fissure. Also type of analgesia was studied, without observe influence of the epidural one on the incidence of anal lesions.

In addition other authors showed that anal fissure was associated with heavier babies, long second stage labour and anal incontinence after delivery. Thus these last results suggested that traumatic delivery, although it's an important risk factor, should not be considered the only cause of postpartum anal fissure.

Several reports during recent years have underlined that resting anal canal pressure is raised in patients with chronic anal fissure. However to date is still uncertain if this represents a primary abnormality or it's a secondary response to sphincter irritation.

During the puerperium women may have a reduction of anal canal pressures after vaginal delivery.

To investigate the role of anal sphincter hypertonia in the etiology of postpartum anal fissures, Corby et al. evaluated the effect of parturition on the pelvic floor in primigravid women. They found that antenatal mean maximum resting and squeeze increment anal canal pressures were no different in women who did and in those who did not develop anal fissure. Six weeks after delivery, mean maximum resting and squeeze increment pressures fell in both groups compared with antenatal values. This highlights that anal canal sphincter hypertonia is not a primary phenomenon in postpartum anal fissure, and that anal canal pressures are significantly reduced in the puerperium [35]. Accordingly it is conceivable a different physiopathology of anal fissure during pregnancy.

Treatment of anal fissure during childbirth and postpartum period is aimed at avoiding constipation and relieving internal sphincter spasm. Laxative and high-fiber diet with psyllium seed supplementation are recommended; iron preparations should be temporarily discontinued. Locally applied lidocaine ointment can be effective, and warm water soaks help relieve anal sphincter spasm. Literature data show that this treatment is frequently successful.

Those who fail to respond to these conservative measures are candidates for surgical procedures.

Anal dilatation and lateral internal sphincterotomy, the conventional surgical approach to chronic anal fissure, are based on the assumption that either primary or secondary anal sphincter hypertonia prevents internal sphincter relaxation during defecation, perpetuating a cycle of injury and spasm. Both precedures carry unpredictable risks of faecal incontinence. Some authors showed that postpartum anal fissure is not associated with increased anal canal pressure, rather than pressures are significantly reduced postpartum. Besides vaginal delivery may potentially cause anal canal injury. In this situation further surgical damage to the anal sphincter mechanisms clearly risks incontinence. For these reasons most colorectal surgeon are reluctant to perform lateral internal sphincterotomy. In seeking to avoid this complication seems more prudent use other kind of therapy, like topical glycerine trinitrate, botulinum toxin or advancement flaps, without interference to the internal anal sphincter.

CONCLUSION

In the assessment of the patient with diagnosis of anal fissure, the physician always has to keep in mind the possibility of particular cases. The identification of such coexisting pathologies, as underlined in this chapter, implies an appropriate therapeutic choice to avoid injuries to patients.

The primary endpoint is to obtain healing by a conservative medical treatment; however if this therapy fails, surgery seems to be safe and feasible.

These kinds of patients request a tailored surgery to decrease the risks of postoperative complications.

REFERENCES

[1] Collins E, Lund J. A review of chronic anal fissure management. *Tech. Colonproctol.*, 2007; 11:209-223.
[2] Lund JN, Scholefield JH. Aetiology and treatment of anal fissure. *Br. J. Surg.*, 1996; 83:1335-1344.
[3] Hananel N, Gordon PH. Re-examination of clinical manifestations and response to therapy of fissure in ano. *Dis. Colon Rectum*, 1997; 40:229-233.
[4] Madoff R, Fleshman J. AGA technical Review on the Diagnosis and Care of Patients With Anal Fissure. *Gastroenterology*, 2003; 124:235-245.
[5] Schwartz DA, Loftus EV Jr. The natural history of fistulizing Crohn's disease in Olmsted County, Minnesota. *Gastroenterology*, 2002; 122:875-80.
[6] Lewis RT, Maron DJ. Anorectal Crohn's disease. *Surg. Clin. North Am.* 2010;90:83-97.
[7] Beaugerie L, Seksik P et al. Predictors of Crohn's disease. *Gastroenterology,* 2006; 130:650-6.

[8] Gelbmann CM, Rogler G et al. Prior bowel resections, perianal disease, and a high initial Crohn's disease activity index are associated with corticosteroid resistance in active Crohn's disease. *Am. J. Gastroenterol.*, 2002; 97:1438-45.
[9] Sweeney JL, Ritchie JK, Nicholls RJ. Anal fissure in Crohn's disease. *Br. J. Surg.*, 1988; 75:56-7.
[10] Fleshner PR, Schoetz DJ Jr et al. Anal fissure in Crohn's disease: a plea for aggressive management. *Dis. Colon Rectum,* 1995; 38:1137-1143.
[11] Sangwan YP, Schoetz DJ Jr et al. Perianal Crohn's disease: results of local surgical treatment. *Dis. Colon Rectum*, 1996; 39:529-35.
[12] Makowiec F, Jehle EC, Starlinger M. Clinical course of perianal fistulas in Crohn's disease. *Gut.*, 1995; 37:696-701.
[13] Sandborn WJ, Fazio VW et al. AGA technical review on perianal Crohn's disease. *Gastroenterology,* 2003; 125:1508-30.
[14] Palder SB, Shandling B et al. Perianal complications of pediatric Crohn's disease. *J. Pediatr. Surg.,* 1991; 26:513-5.
[15] Cosnes J, Cattan S et al. Long-term evolution of disease behavior of Crohn's disease. *Inflamm. Bowel Dis.,* 2002; 8:244-50.
[16] Singh B, Mortensen NJ et al. Perianal Crohn's disease. *British Journal of Surgery,* 2004; 91:801-814.
[17] Barrett WL, Callahan TD, Orkin BA. Perianal manifestations of human immunodeficiency virus infection: experience with 260 patients. *Dis. Colon Rectum* 1998; 41:606-612.
[18] Wolkomir AF, Luchtefeld MA. Surgery for Symptomatic Hemorrhoids and Anal Fissures in Crohn's Disease. *Dis. Colon Rectum,* 1993; 36:545-547.
[19] Abcarian H. Perianal Crohn's disease. *Semin. Colon Rectal Surg.*, 1994; 5:210-5.
[20] Alexander-Williams J, Buchmann P. Perianal Crohn's disease. *World J. Surg.*, 1980; 4:203-8.
[21] Platell C, Mackay J et al. Anal pathology in patients with Crohn's disease. *Aust. N. Z. J. Surg.,* 1996; 66:5-9.
[22] Steele SR. Operative management of Crohn's disease of the colon including anorectal disease. *Surg. Clin. North Am.,* 2007; 87:611-31.
[23] McClane SJ, Rombeau JL. Anorectal Crohn's disease. *Surg. Clin. North Am.,* 2001; 81:169-183.
[24] Wolkomir AF, Luchtefeld MA. Surgery for symptomatic hemorrhoids and anal fissures in Crohn's disease. *Dis. Colon Rectum,* 1993; 36:545-547.
[25] Allan A, Keighley MR. Management of perianal Crohn's disease. *World J. Surg.,* 1988; 12:198-202.

[26] Miles AJ, Mellor CH et al. Surgical management of anorectal disease in HIV-positive homosexuals. *Br. J. Surg.,* 1990; 77:869-71.
[27] Carr ND, Mercey D, Slack WW. Non-condylomatous, perianal disease in homosexual men. *Br. J. Surg.,* 1989; 76:1064-6.
[28] Burke EC, Orloff SL et al. Wound healing after anorectal surgery in human immunodeficiency virus-infected patients. *Arch. Surg.,* 1991; 126:1267-70.
[29] Hammer SM, Squires KE et al. A controlled trial of two nucleoside analogue plus indinavir in persons with HIV infection and CD4 cell counts of 200 cubic millimeter or less. *N. Engl. J. Med.*, 1997; 337:725-33.
[30] Weiss EG, Wexner SD. Surgery for anal lesions in HIV infected patients. *Ann. Med.,* 1995; 27:467-75.
[31] Schmitt SL, Wexner SD. Treatment of anorectal manifestations of AIDS: past and present. *Int. J. STD AIDS*, 1994; 5:8-10.
[32] Lord RV. Anorectal surgery in patients infected with human immunodeficiency virus: factors associated with delayed wound healing. *Ann. Surg.,* 1997; 226:92-9.
[33] Viamonte M, Dailey TH, Gottesman L. Ulcerative disease of the anorectum in the HIV+ patient. *Dis. Colon Rectum,* 1993; 36:801-5.
[34] Consten EC, Slors FJ et al. Anorectal surgery in human immunodeficiency virus-infected patients. Clinical outcome in relation to immune status. *Dis. Colon Rectum,* 1995; 38:1169-75.
[35] Corby H, Donnelly VS et al. Anal canal pressures are low in women with postpartum anal fissure. *Br. J. Surg.,* 1997; 84:86-8.
[36] Abramowitz L, Sobhani I et al. Anal fissure and thrombosed external hemorrhoids before and after delivery. *Dis Colon Rectum,* 2002; 45:650-5.
[37] Abramowitz L, Batallan A. Epidemiology of anal lesions (fissure and thrombosed external hemorroid) during pregnancy and post-partum. *Gynecol. Obstet. Fertil.,* 2003; 31:546-9.
[38] Medich DS, Fazio VW. Hemorrhoids, anal fissure, and carcinoma of the colon, rectum, and anus during pregnancy. *Surg. Clin. North Am.,* 1995; 75:77-88.
[39] Calhoun BC. Gastrointestinal disorders in pregnancy. *Obstet. Gynecol. Clin. North Am.,* 1992; 19:733-44.
[40] Martin JD. Postpartum anal fissure. *Lancet.* 1953; 1:271-3.

In: Anal Fissure
Editors: P. Sileri and A. L. Gaspari
ISBN: 978-1-61209-716-9
© 2012 Nova Science Publishers, Inc

Chapter 7

CONSERVATIVE AND SURGICAL TREATMENT OF CHRONIC ANAL FISSURE: LONGER-TERM RESULTS FROM OUR PROSPECTIVE DATABASE

Luana Franceschilli, Giulio P. Angelucci, Sara Lazzaro, Alessandra Di Giorgio, Achille L. Gaspari and Pierpaolo Sileri[1].
University of Rome
Tor Vergata, Policlinico Tor Vergata, Rome, Italy

INTRODUCTION

The treatment of chronic anal fissure (CAF) has changed greatly during the past two decades with ongoing research on medical approaches directed at lowering the internal anal sphincter tone, and avoiding the risk of faecal continence disturbance. Glycerin trinitrate (GTN), topical calcium channel blockers and anal dilatation and botulinum toxin injection alone are all known to be able to lower the IAS tone but results have been disappointing in curing CAF, often marginally better than to placebo.

In a recent meta-analysis of randomized clinical trials comparing medical treatments to placebo or surgery [1], Nelson et al. have shown that GNT,

---

[1] Corresponding author: Pierpaolo Sileri, University of Rome Tor Vergata, Policlinico Tor Vergata, Chirurgia generale (6B) Viale Oxford 81, 00133, Rome, Italy. Ph +390620902927; +390620902926, email: piersileri@yahoo.com.

botulinum toxin injection, and surgery have overall response rates of about 55%, 65%, and 85%, respectively, whereas the placebo healing rate is about 35% across all the studies. This evidence led Nichols in a recent editorial to point out that surgery in the form of sphincterotomy is markedly superior to any form of chemical sphincterotomy and is the most effective treatment for fissure at present [2].

Lateral internal sphincterotomy (LIS) allows prompt healing in more than over 90% of the patients with a very low recurrence risk of 3%. However it may cause minor but permanent incontinence [3-10]. According to a systematic review of randomized surgical trials [11], the overall risk of continence disturbance after surgery is about 10% but can be as high as 35% from non prospective non controlled data.

Obviously these findings augment the fear of incontinence and reluctance toward surgery for both the patient and the surgeon with the continuing call for changes to safe medical alternatives.

Medical treatment seems therefore a reasonable first line therapy for most patients with CAF. Second line use of botulinum toxin seems to heal only 50% of fissures resistant to [12]. It is likely that the fibrotic nature of chronic fissures resistant to GTN is not resolved by chemical sphincterotomy alone. Fissurectomy alone is not currently used in adults, but its combination with botulinum toxin injection has been recently used with success to treat fissures resistant to medical treatment [13,14,15], with healing rates higher than 90%, not far from LIS and with negligible risk of incontinence.

We have previously demonstrated that surgical treatment either with fissurectomy and botulinum toxin injection and LIS is safe and associated with the highest likelihood of CAF healing compared to common medical treatments. However, we concluded that despite LIS may be appropriately offered without a trial of pharmacological treatment, being incontinence a lifelong risk, a step-wise approach should be offered starting with medical treatment for high risk patients. Hence we proposed Botulinum injections and Fissurectomy as rational, safe and effective first line treatment. In this prospective study we present longer-term results in a larger cohort of patients with CAF assessing the efficacy of different conservative treatments (including GTN and anal dilators or a combination of the two) and surgery.

PATIENTS AND METHODS

Between January 2004 and July 2010, 423 consecutive patients with CAF and with complete follow-up were enrolled in the study. Diagnosis was made according to history and physical exam. CAF was defined by duration of symptoms longer than three months and the presence of a skin tag, a sentinel pile or fibrosis at the margins of the fissure. Exclusion criteria included atypical CAF associated with grade III/IV haemorrhoids, previous anal surgery, incontinence, inflammatory bowel disease, infection or cancer. Patients with coexisting medical conditions requiring calcium channel blockers and oral, sublingual or transdermal nitrates were also considered ineligible for this study. Patients with incomplete follow-up or lost were also excluded.

During the outpatient visit a complete explanation of the disease as well as the medical treatment options, benefits and side effects were given to the patient.

After this, each patient was assigned to an eight-week course of medical therapy with either 0.2% GTN or anal dilators (DIL) according to his/her preference. Patients in the GTN group were instructed to apply the ointment twice a day to the edge and just inside the anal canal (morning and evening) after a warm Sitz bath. The amount of crème to be applied was shown during the outpatient visit. If patients experienced side effects, he was instructed to use a finger glove for application or to reduce the amount to be applied.

Patients of DIL group were instructed to use an anal dilators set (Dilatan, Sapi Med, Alessandria, Italy) as follows. In order to ease the DIL introduction, after heated for 15 minutes in water, patients lubricated the DIL with a preparation gel (Dilatan crema, Sapi Med, Alessandria, Italy) and introduced it fully into the anal canal, and maintained the position for 10 minutes twice a day (morning and evening). Patient was invited to repeat this procedure for 3 weeks starting with small diameter dilators (20-23 mm), followed by medium size dilators (23-27 mm) and ending with the large (30 mm). An illustrated brochure containing practical suggestions was given to the patient.

The primary end-point was fissure healing at last follow-up. Secondary end-points were symptomatic improvement, need for surgery, side effects and surgical complications, and patients' satisfaction.

Improvement was defined as absence of pain or bleeding. Healing was defined as complete epithelialization of the fissure base. Those patients in which no improvement in symptoms was observed after 8 weeks were crossed to the other treatment (either GTN or DIL) or switched to a combination of the two for additional 4 weeks according to his/her preference. Botulinum toxin injection in the IAS associated to fissurectomy (BTX-F) or lateral internal sphyncterotomy

(LIS) were offered to patients who did not benefit from the 12-weeks treatment course with GTN or DIL or a combination of them, after full information about the risks and the benefits of either procedure. Patients with non-healed or recurrent CAF who refused surgery were offered a further medical treatment. Anorectal manometry was performed before either one of the procedures.

Either fissurectomy/Botox injection or LIS were performed in a day-surgery setting under sedation and local anaesthesia in lithotomy position. Before surgery, all patients had a limited bowel preparation with one Sorbiclis (Sofar S.p.a, Milan, Italy). An Eisenhammer speculum was gently inserted, avoiding excessive sphincter dilatation. Fissurectomy was always performed by minimal excision of the fibrotic edges of the fissure and curettage of its base just back to fresh, normal, non fibrotic tissue. If present, the sentinel pile was excised with cutting diathermy. Once fissurectomy was performed, 25 units of botulinum toxin (Botox, Allergan, Milan, Italy) were injected as follows. A volume of 1.6 ml of saline solution was mixed into a 100-unit vial of botulinum toxin and 0.4 ml aliquot (equal to 25 units) was drawn up into a 1 ml syringe with a 27 Gauge needle and injected equally into the IAS at 3 and 9 o'clock.

An open LIS was performed with patient in lithotomic position under local anaesthesia and deep sedation when necessary. A circumanal incision of 1 cm was made just distal to the inter-sphincteric grove in the lateral position with subsequent partial division of the internal anal sphincter using coagulation diathermy. The distal internal sphincter was divided under direct vision for a length up to the fissure apex. In all cases fissurectomy was performed as previously described [14].

Patients in both groups were discharged home on the same day and stayed on a high residue diet and stool softener for 7 days. A non narcotic analgesic was also prescribed as needed and patients were advised to take regular warm sitz baths. Patients were seen in outpatient clinic after 1 week and therefore at 1- 2- 3- and 12-month intervals. Patients were then contacted by phone. Independently of these scheduled appointments, patients were seen on request. Information about fissure healing, symptoms, complications and adverse effects were prospectively collected. Wexner incontinence score was used to assess continence after the procedures.

Differences between treatment groups were evaluated by chi square test.

RESULTS

Patients' demographics, fissure characteristics and treatment failures are shown in table 1.

Table 1. Patients' demographics, fissure characteristics and treatment failures

	GTN	DIL	GTN/DIL	BOTOX/ fissurectomy	LIS
Number (N)	289	134	51	38	83
Mean Age (years)	46	45	47	39	45
Sex M/F	149/140	61/73	18/33	14/24	36/47
Fissure position					
Posterior	257	112	33	34	70
Anterior	24	18	13	3	10
Both/ other	8	4	5	1	3
Sentinel pile N/%	121/289 42.9%	88/134 65.7%	33/51 64.7%	23/38 60.5%	54/83 65.1%
Single treatment (12 weeks) success N/(%)	187/289 (64.7%)	83/134 (61.9%)	NA	NA	NA
Recurrence	29/187 (15.5%)	8/83 (9.6%)	NA	NA	NA
After cross-over healing N/%	24/54 (44.4%)	24/41 (58.5%)	20/51 (39.2%)	NA	NA
Recurrence	4/24 (16.6%)	3/24 (12.5%)	4/20 (20%)	NA	NA
Overall Success N/%	178/289 (61.6%)	96/134 (71.6%)	16/51 (31.4%)	32/38 (84.2%)	82/83 (98.8%)
Overall Success N/% (DIL/GTN combined included)	186/289 (64.4%)	100/134 (74.6%)	NA	NA	88/89 (98.9%)

GTN: nitroglycerin ointment; DIL: anal dilators; BTX: botulinum; LIS: lateral internal sphincterotomy. NA: not applicable.

Median follow-up was 36 +/-17 months ranging from 3 to 78 months.

Healing after 12 weeks was observed in 64.7% (187/289) of the patients for the GTN only group and in 61.9% (83/134) of the patients for the DIL only group without significant differences (p=0.3). Overall fissure healing after medical treatment with either GTN or DIL alone was observed in a total of 270 (63.8%) patients.

Recurrence rate after 12 weeks treatment was 15.5% for GTN only group and 9.6% for DIL only group respectively (p=0.02) reducing the overall healing rate of single medical treatment to 55.0% (233 patients).

In particular, healing with no recurrence was observed in 158 out of 289 patients (54.6%) treated with GTN alone and in 75 out of 134 patients (55.9%) who underwent anal dilation only. In most of the patients, healing time ranged from 8 to 12 weeks after treatment course. No significant difference was noted between the two groups in terms of time to healing .

One hundred-forty-six patients (34.5%) experienced non-healing or sudden recurring disease during the first 8 weeks observation period. Of those, 54 patients (previously treated with GTN) were switched to DIL, 41 (previously treated with DIL) to GTN for additional 4 weeks. The remaining 59 patients accepted a combined GTN/DIL treatment.

A total 68 patients (16.1%) responded to this further medical therapy and overall definitive healing rate rose significantly to 68.7% (p=0.001). In particular, at the end of this further 4 weeks treatment, GTN after DIL resulted effective in 58.5% of the treated patients (24 out 41) and DIL after GTN in 44.4% (24 out of 54) (p=0.4). Of the 51 patients treated with combined DIL/GTN, 20 responded with healing (35.2%) (p=0.6 vs DIL and p=0.09 vs GTN). During the follow-up recurrence rates were 16.6% for DIL after GTN, 12.5% for GTN after DIL, and 20% for combined GTN/DIL, with no significant differences among groups.

Definitive healing was observed in 20 out of 54 patients treated with DIL after GTN (37.0%), in 21 out of 41 patients treated with GTN after DIL (51.2%) and in 16 out of 51 patients treated with combined GTN/DIL (31.3%). DIL after GTN and combined GTN/DIL treatments were similar in terms of definitive healing but worse compared GTN after DIL treatment although difference did not appear significant (p=0.06).

At the end of the study, overall medical treatment (including the cross-over) success was 64.4% and 74.6% respectively for patients initially treated with GTN or DIL. This difference between the two groups was statistically significant (p=0.01). At the end of the study 68.7% of the patients resulted cured by medical approach alone.

Overall incidence of GTN side effects was 8.9% (28 out of 313 patients), mostly mild headache (20 patients) and pruritus ani (8 patients). Seven patients (2.2%) discontinued therapy and were switched to DIL.

A total of 226 patients were treated with DIL (134 patients as initial treatment and 92 patients after GTN treatment) and 9.3% interrupted the DIL course because of severe discomfort. After non-healing or recurrence, surgery was offered to 116 patients (27.4%). At the end of follow-up eight patients refused either botulinum treatment or surgery and further medical treatment was offered with minimal beneficial effect. Of the remaining 121 patients, 38 underwent Fissurectomy/Botox injection and 83 to LIS. Healing was reported in 32 out of 38 (84.2%) patients after fissurectomy/Botox injection. This percentage was significantly higher compared to GTN alone course (p=0.001), to DIL alone treatment (p=0.004) or to overall combined/cross-over groups (p=0.001). One patient (2.6%) experienced transitory flatus incontinence. Non-healing was observed in 2 patients (5.2%) and recurrence in 4 (10.5%). Despite reluctance to further surgery after failed fissurectomy/botox by two patients, all 4 patients underwent LIS had complete healing. No perioperative complications were observed in this group.

All but one patient treated with LIS showed complete healing with no postoperative incontinence. Overall morbidity after LIS was 7.8%. Three patients experienced urinary retention after surgery (all males) and needed catheterization. Two patients experienced perianal ecchymosis and one perianal abscess with submucosal fistula that required surgery 7 months later. One patient experienced recurrence 10 months after surgery.

Comparing the different treatment groups, there were no significant differences in terms of healing rates between males and females, presence or absence of sentinel pile or previous GTN or/and DIL treatment.

DISCUSSION

The most recent theories on etiopathogenesis of anal fissures have focused on increased tonicity of the IAS, which induces ischaemia of the anodermis mainly of the posterior commissure.

IAS contains smooth muscle fibers whose contraction is controlled by neural influences and myogenic mechanisms [16,17] and increased cytosol calcium levels mediate its contraction. Nitric oxide serves as the main neurotransmitter in the IAS causing relaxation of the muscle fibers [17]. Numerous clinical evidences pointed out the role of an elevated resting pressure of the IAS in patients with anal fissures [18,19]. Factors causing IAS hypertonia are not well understood but a significant role in perpetuating the muscle spasm is played by the trauma caused by the passage of hard stools on the mucosa [20]. Spasm of the sphincter not only promotes constipation (thus setting up a vicious cycle) but also leads to compression of the terminal arterioles supplying the mucosa of the anal canal [21]. Impaired blood flow in this already poorly perfused area prevents fissure healing. This is why chronic anal fissure has been described as an ischemic ulcer [22].

Since the introduction of the posterior internal sphincterotomy by Eisenhammer in 1951, CAF has been managed with surgery once conservative measures failed [23]. The more safe lateral sphincterotomy, popularized by Notaras in 1969, has until recently been the mainstay of treatment in order to reduce the pathologically raised pressure profile within the anal canal [24]. Despite surgery is highly efficacious and succeeds in curing CAF in more than 90% of patients (often exceeds 95% with high patient satisfaction), postoperative impairment of continence is not uncommon [1,17]. The incidence is not well documented and varies between 0 and 35% for flatus incontinence, 0 and 21% for liquid incontinence, and 0 and 5% for solid stool incontinence [25-28]. As indicated by Nelson in a recent systematic review of randomized surgical trials, the overall risk of incontinence is about 10% [1,11,29], mostly to flatus without any specification of the duration of this problem (transitory or permanent). However, it is a common believe that the risk of permanent incontinence is approximately 1-3%. In 2005, Casillas et al conducted a review of patients who had undergone LIS for a fissure, comparing a postal survey response of these patients to hospital notes [30]. Chart review revealed incontinence to stool and gas as 2.8% and 4.4%, respectively, whereas the postal survey of the same group of patients revealed the incidences to be 28.7% and 31.5% [30]. Surgeons consequently may significantly underestimate the scale of postoperative impairment of continence following LIS in less anonymous follow-up techniques are used [31]. Nonetheless, this does not take into account normal weakening of the sphincter with age as well as the possibility of future anorectal surgery, radiation or obstetrical trauma. So, the risk of incontinence after LIS should be considered lifelong, to an often young, otherwise healthy person. Besides endoanal ultrasound reports demonstrate extensive permanent sphincter defects in patients after LIS even if the patient remains continent [27]. As well as the destruction of the IAS, other possible causes have been proposed. In one study, patients incontinent following LIS were noted to have a thinner external sphincter than those who were continent postoperatively [32].

In order to minimize this risk, several authors have tried a more limited division of internal sphincter, a tailored or controlled sphincterotomy, but additional persuasive data is needed [33,34].

Nonetheless, in addition to continence disturbance, general surgical complications rate has been reported to range from 7% to 42% mostly related to hemorrhage, abscess, fistula, faecal impaction and urinary retention [35].

In the late 1990s when alternatives to surgery were sought because of risk of incontinence, costs, and time for recovery newer medications directed at relaxing increased sphincter tone or enhancing mucosal blood flow were investigated. These included nitroglycerin ointment, calcium channel blockers (either given as tablets or topically) and, recently, injection of botulinum toxin.

GTN causes sphincter relaxation by acting as a nitric oxide donor and improves anodermal perfusion [36]. Topical calcium channel blockers like diltiazem and nifedipine induce IAS by decreasing cytosolic calcium concentration.

Despite early trials (including both acute and chronic fissure) of conservative medical treatments showed overall healing rates and pain relief close to surgery, usually results with medical treatments are only marginally better than placebo or conservative therapies alone (fiber, Sitz baths, topical lidocaine) with healing rates between 36% to 68% and relapses rates as high as 35% (37,38). According to Nelson's metanalysis, a marginal advantage in using GTN (55%) over placebo (35%) exists but no statistical difference was found comparing GTN to either botulinum toxin or calcium channel blockers.

We used GTN ointment in addition to conservative approaches (fiber and Sitz bath) as first line treatment because of its safety, convenience and cost. The dosage and number of applications previously reported ranges from 0.2% to 0.5% and from twice to four per day [39,40]. Dose escalation or use of a transdermal patch has not been shown to improve the healing rate [41,42]. The principal side effect is headache, seen in up to 50% of patients, and less commonly anal pruritus [37,43-45]. Hence compliance issues are observed in up to 72% of patients and about 20% of patients will discontinue therapy [29, 42,46].

Since 0.2% dosage seems to be as effective as 0.5% dosage, with fewer side effects, we decided to offer a 0.2% twice a day treatment. Our healing rate after GTN alone treatment was close to 55% increasing to only 62% after cross-over to DIL and to 65% if DIL/GTN combined course is considered. We also observed a 15.5% recurrence rate, similar to combined GTN/DIL, but higher compared to DIL use only (9.6% p=0.01, DIL after GTN 16.6% p=0.5) and GTN after DIL (12.5% p=0.4). These findings did not differ from our previous observations apart a significant lower success of DIL/GTN combined therapy.

In our series the incidence of side effects associated with GTN application was lower (8.9%) than the common incidence of at least 20-30% reported in literature and lower than our previous report (12.8%). Headache is the most commonly reported GTN side effect ranging between 10-72% at a dosage of 0.2%, despite this percentage raises with higher dosage (47). About 2% of the patients discontinued the therapy and were switched to DIL. GTN therapy was discontinued because of headache (**4** patients) and pruritus ani (3 patients). As previously observed, we believe that the low incidence of side effects and good compliance to treatment program showed by our groups of patients is the result of reduced number of applications (twice a day) and the accuracy of instructions given to the patient at the time of the outpatient visit.

The rationale for the use of anal dilators (DIL) is the finding that they induce muscle relaxation with consequent reduction in sphincter hypertonia. Moreover blood flow is improved in the IAS thus favoring fissure healing. When the DIL is heated, the relaxing effect is enhanced [45]. Short-term healing rates are reported as high as 95% when used in combination with GTN (46-49), with about 10% reduction after 2 years follow up. However little evidence on the efficacy of anal dilators is present in the literature. Recently, Schiano et al. reported healing rates of 75% with DIL only and 93.7% with combined GTN/DIL treatment [45]. In our experience the DIL-only treatment was associated with a 55.9% healing rate, significantly superior to GTN use only (41.8%). The significantly lower recurrence rate after DIL alone (9.6% versus 15.5%) may explain this result. It seems that DIL use allows a durable healing and the reduced recurrence rates observed when DIL is implemented (either added or as switch after GTN) may suggest this observation. This observation is confirmed by the observed success rates at the end of the study: 65.9% for initially treated with GTN versus 74.6% for initially treated with DIL (significant difference). It may argued that patients initially treated with dilatation experienced less pain as expression of less severe disease at the time of diagnosis thus more likely to agree for such treatment and with more chances to heal. As a matter of fact, patients who decided for DIL instead of GTN treatment presented a lower visual analogue scale (VAS) score at presentation despite this trend was not statistically significant.

When DIL group was switched to GTN because of non-healing, the success rate increased not significantly, than the success rate observed when GTN course was followed by DIL. We explain this difference with a shorter healing time observed with GTN compared to DIL course that needs few weeks applications of different size dilators. A 4 weeks DIL course may not be sufficient to significantly increase the healing rate after GTN thus reducing the likelihood of surgery. This result is far from the 93.5% healing rate, reported by Schiano et al. Our longer follow up may temper this difference. In our experience DIL use is safe, healing rate are slightly better to GTN treatment, but compliance is lower. Overall 9.3% of the patients (versus 2.2% of GTN) interrupted the DIL course because of severe discomfort preferring "less invasive" approaches. The reluctance in using DIL after GTN failure (either as crossover or in combination) as well as the reduced compliance may explain the low healing rate observed in this group.

In the recent years, injection of botulinum toxin A into the internal sphincter has emerged as an alternative to surgery in the treatment of CAF. By a temporary chemical sphincterotomy it allows fissure healing in approximately 50% of resistant CAF when used alone and as much as 93% in the short and medium term when combined to fissurectomy [50].

The botulinum toxin is believed to act at the postganglionic level reducing noradrenaline output from sympathetic neural terminals in the internal sphincter and possibly also by reducing myogenic tone in this tissue [34]. A single botulinum injection is well tolerated, with minor side effects thus eliminating non compliance issues. It reduces maximum resting pressure by a similar proportion to that of GTN (25-30%) [46], but muscle paralysis occurs within hours after injection and the effect remains over a 2-3 months period of time [25, 51]. Botulinum injection is a simple procedure, easy to learn and can be also done in the outpatient clinic without the need for sedation or local anesthesia.

The most common side effect is transient incontinence to flatus (up to 10%) or feces (up to 5%) [48], which may persist until the toxin's effect have worn off by neuronal degeneration [52]. To date there is only one case of long-term faecal incontinence after botulinum injection [53].

Recurrence are common, but may be easily treated with a good rate of healing even if up to 20% of patients will need LIS [29,49, 54].

There is no consensus on dose, site or number of injections [55]. However a dosage between 20 and 25 units and anterior injection seems more effective and causes no additional side effects [16,17,44]. A transient decrease in mean squeeze pressure can also be observed when higher doses are used [48,56]. Conversely, higher doses are not proven to be more effective [57].

Despite early trials have shown healing rates as high as 90% for acute and chronic fissures, the enthusiasm was tempered by the disappointing results on CAF. Lindsey et al. in a prospective study of 40 patients with GTN-resistant fissures treated with 20 units of botulinum, reported an healing rate of only 43% [12]. Similarly Minguez et al. [58] did not show healing rates as high as surgery after botulinum injection with a 42 months follow up, while Arroyo and Mentes observed 1-year recurrence rates after botulinum injection approaching respectively 50% and 40% [59,60]. Higher healing rates are observed if botulinum is given early, before the chronic fibrosis of the fissure is established [46]. Since botulinum injection treats only the internal sphincter spasm, Lindsey et al have proposed to add fissurectomy to chemical sphincterotomy reporting a healing rate of 93% for medically resistant CAF [25]. In a more recent study Scholz reports excellent results with implementation of the fissurectomy-Botox injection technique, which proved to be effective in treating fissure recurrences, too [61].

Fissurectomy enhances healing removing the fibrotic fissure edges, unhealthy granulation tissue at the base and the sentinel pile when present [25]. Fissurectomy alone creates in essence an acute fissure with fresh wound edges, but does not address the underlying IAS spasm at the base of CAF pathogenesis. Few authors suggested that higher rates of fissure healing could be achieved if fissurectomy is combined with conservative pharmacological sphincterotomy [31].

We adopted this novel sphincter-sparing procedure as second line treatment after failure of GTN and/or DIL course. We observed a long term healing rate of 83.3%, significantly higher than the one reported after all other medical approaches. Along with Lindsey et al, we believe that fissure healing is significantly higher with fissurectomy-botulinum toxin injection compared to medical treatment alone, because with this treatment we are able to address both elements of chronic fissure, chronic fibrosis and internal sphincter spasm. We observed a single case of transitory low grade incontinence (Wexner Incontinence Score=2), but our data confirm the safety of this treatment. The main drawback of this approach is the need of an operating theater and the costs. Although 5 patients of this group experienced fissure recurrence or non-healing, with all requiring subsequent LIS at certain point, fissurectomy and botulinum injection reduces significantly the need of LIS. The paucity of minor side effects associated to the good healing rates indicate that Botulinum injection/fissurectomy may be used as first line approach for selected CAF even without previous medical treatment. Along with Lindsey et al, our study confirms that medical treatment alone for chronic, well-established fissures might be inappropriate, merely delaying definitive fissure healing [14]. Features of chronic fissure such as a fibrotic tissue, skin tag or sentinel pile predict poor healing with medical therapy and disappointing results of medical therapies for CAF, often similar, or just superior to placebo in different clinical trials, strengthen this observation.

As a consequence of our experience and literature evidence, we believe that BTX/fissurectomy should be offered as first line treatment for patients with typical CAF even without previous medical/conservative treatments. Patients at high risk for anal incontinence, young female patients, patients with previous anal surgery can also be treated with BTX/fissurectomy. Botulinum toxin injection associated to a gentle fissurectomy seems to be very safe, reducing greatly the likelihood of surgery and abolishing the risk of incontinence. The main drawback of BTX/fissurectomy is the need of surgery and the costs. However, we believe that the prompt and excellent healing rates (close to LIS), the absence of severe side effects or complications might justify the costs.

Failure of BTX/fissurectomy or recurrence indicates the need of LIS.

Our study confirms that LIS represents the most effective approach to CAF with minor morbidity and minimal recurrence rate. Although transitory postoperative incontinence can been observed in up to one third of patients, in our experience we did not incur in any. Nonetheless we did not observe any permanent incontinence.

Our general complication rate after LIS was approximately 18% within the range reported from the literature [35].

Although the proximal extent of the LIS continue to be a topic of debate, in our experience, by 'tailoring' the amount of sphincter to be divided to the length of the fissure, the risk of incontinence is minimized as well as the fissure healing achieved.

The proximal extent of LIS up to the apex of fissure, although associated with a slower healing and increased risk of recurrence [16, 35, 61], allows a minimal risk of continence disturbance as observed in our study. Proximal extent of LIS is particularly important in female patients, because of the shorter length of the internal sphincter and vaginal deliveries that have been found to a be a significant risk factor of incontinence after LIS [30].

To overcome the risk of slower healing and recurrence with a conservative or 'tailored LIS', we believe that an accurate fissurectomy should always be added to LIS as previously discussed.

In conclusion, although LIS is far more effective than medical treatments, BTX injection/fissurectomy as first line treatment may significantly increase the healing rate compared to standard conservative treatment. Moreover this approach as first line treatment allows a faster healing time compared to medical treatments while avoiding any risk of incontinence if compared to LIS.

REFERENCES

[1] Nelson R. Non surgical therapy for anal fissure. *Cochrane Database Syst. Rev.* 2006;(4):CD003431.

[2] Nicholls J. Anal fissure; surgery is the most effective treatment. *Colorectal Dis*. 2008 Jul;10(6):529-30.

[3] Marby M, Alexander-Williams J, Buchmann P, Arabi Y, Kappas A, Minervini S, Gatehouse D, Keighley MR. A randomized controlled trial to compare anal dilatation with lateral subcutaneous sphincterotomy for anal fissure. *Dis. Colon Rectum*. 1979;22:308-11.

[4] Weaver RM, Ambrose NS, Alexander-Williams J, Keighley MR. Manual dilatation of the anus vs. lateral subcutaneous sphincterotomy in the

treatment of chronic fissure-in-ano. Results of a prospective, randomized, clinical trial. *Dis. Colon Rectum*. 1987;30:420-3.
[5] Boulos PB, Araujo JG. Adequate internal sphincterotomy for chronic anal fissure: subcutaneous or open technique? *Br. J. Surg*. 1984;71:360-2.
[6] Jensen SL, Lund F, Nielsen OV, Tange G. Lateral subcutaneous sphincterotomy versus anal dilatation in the treatment of fissure in ano in outpatients: a prospective randomised study. *Br. Med. J.* (Clin. Res. Ed.). 1984;289:528-30.
[7] Kortbeek JB, Langevin JM, Khoo RE, Heine JA. Chronic fissure-in-ano: a randomized study comparing open and subcutaneous lateral internal sphincterotomy. *Dis. Colon Rectum*. 1992;35:835-7.
[8] Wiley M, Day P, Rieger N, Stephens J, Moore J. Open vs. closed lateral internal sphincterotomy for idiopathic fissure-in-ano: a prospective, randomized, controlled trial. *Dis. Colon Rectum*. 2004;47:847-52.
[9] Arroyo A, Perez F, Serrano P, Candela F, Calpena R. Open versus closed lateral sphincterotomy performed as an outpatient procedure under local anesthesia for chronic anal fissure: prospective randomized study of clinical and manometric longterm results. *J. Am. Coll. Surg.* 2004 Sep;199(3):361-7.
[10] Aysan E, Aren A, Ayar E. A prospective, randomized, controlled trial of primary wound closure after lateral internal sphincterotomy. *Am. J. Surg*. 2004;187:291-4.
[11] Nelson R. Operative procedures for fissure in ano. *Cochrane Database Syst. Rev*. 2005;(2):CD002199.
[12] Lindsey I, Jones OM, Cunningham C, George BD, Mortensen NJ. Botulinum toxin as second-line therapy for chronic anal fissure failing 0.2 percent glyceryl trinitrate. *Dis. Colon Re*ctum. 2003;46:361-6.
[13] Scholz T, Hetzer FH, Dindo D, Demartines N, Clavien PA, Hahnloser D. Long-term follow-up after combined fissurectomy and Botox injection for chronic anal fissures. *Int. J. Colorectal Dis*. 2007 Jan 30; [Epub ahead of print]
[14] Lindsey I, Cunningham C, Jones OM, Francis C, Mortensen NJ. Fissurectomy-botulinum toxin: a novel sphincter-sparing procedure for medically resistant chronic anal fissure. *Dis. Colon Rectum*. 2004;47:1947-52.
[15] Sileri P, Mele A, Stolfi VM, Grande M, Sega G, Gentileschi P, Di Carlo S, Gaspari AL. Medical and surgical treatment of chronic anal fissure: a prospective study. *J. Gastrointest. Surg*. 2007 Nov;11(11):1541-8.
[16] Steele S.R., Madoff R.D. Systematic review: the treatment of anal fissure. *Aliment Pharmacol. Ther*. 2006 Jul 15;24(2):247-57.Review.

[17] Ayantunde AA, Debrah SA. Current Concepts in anal Fissures. *World J. Surg.* 2006 Dec;30(12):2246-60.
[18] Lund JN, Binch C., McGrath J., Sparrow RA, Scholefield JH. Topographical distribution of blood supply to the anal canal. *Br. J. Surg.* 1999; 86:496-8.
[19] Klosterhalfen B., Vogel P., Roxen H., Mittermayer C. Topography of the inferior rectal artery: a possible cause of chronic primary anal fissure. *Dis. Colon rectum* 1999;32:43-52.
[20] Lindsey I, Cunningham C, Jones OM, Francis C, Mortensen NJ. Fissurectomy-botulinum toxin: a novel sphincter-sparing procedure for medically resistant chronic anal fissure. *Dis. Colon Rectum* 2004 ;47 :1643-9.
[21] Hancock BD. The internal sphincter and anal fissure. Br. J. Surg. 1977 ; 64 :216-220. *Surg. Gynecol. Obstet*. 1959;109:583.
[22] Schouten WR, Briel JW, Auwerda JJ. Relationship between anal pressure and anodermal blood flow. The vascular pathogenesis of anal fissures. *Dis. Colon Rectum.* 1994 Jul;37(7):664-9.
[23] Eisenhammer S. The evaluation of the internal anal sphincterotomy operation with special reference to anal fissure. *Gynecol. Obstet* 1959; 109:583.
[24] Notaras MJ. Lateral subcutaneous sphincterotomy for anal fissure- a new technique. *J. R. Soc. Med*. 1969;62:713.
[25] Lindsey I, Cunningham C, Jones OM, Francis C, Mortensen NJ. Fissurectomy-botulinum toxin: a novel sphincter-sparing procedure for medically resistant chronic anal fissure. *Dis. Colon Rectum* 2004 Nov;47(11):1947-52.
[26] Nyam DC, Pemberton JH. Long-term results of lateral internal sphincterotomy for chronic anal fissure with particular reference to incidence of fecal incontinence. *Dis. Colon Rectum* 1999;42:1306-10.
[27] Sultan AH, Kamm MA,Nicholls RJ, Bartram CI. Prospective study of the extent of internal anal sphincter division during lateral internal sphincterotomy. *Dis. Colon Rectum* 1994;37:1291-5.
[28] Khubchandani IT, Reed JF. Sequelae of internal sphincterotomy for chronic fissure-in-ano. *Br. J. Surg*. 1989;76:431-4.
[29] Orsay C, Rakinic J, Perry WB, Hyman N, Buie D, et al. Practice parameters for the Management of anal Fissures (Revised). *Dis. Colon Rectum* 2004 Dec ;47(12) :2003-7.

[30] Casillas S, Hull TL, Zutshi M, Trzcinski R, Bast JF, Xu M. Incontinence after a lateral internal sphincterotomy: are we underestimating it? *Dis. Colon Rectum.* 2005 Jun;48(6):1193-9.
[31] Collins EE, Lund JN. A review of chronic anal fissure management. *Tech. Coloproctol.* 2007 Sep;11(3):209-23. Epub 2007 Aug 3. Review.
[32] García-Aguilar J, Belmonte Montes C, Perez JJ, Jensen L, Madoff RD, Wong WD. Incontinence after lateral internal sphincterotomy: anatomic and functional evaluation. *Dis. Colon Rectum.* 1998 Apr;41(4):423-7.
[33] Cho DY. :Controlled Lateral Sphincterotomy for Chronic Anal Fissure. *Dis. Colon Rectum.* 2005 May ;48(5) :1037-41.
[34] Jones OM, Brading AF, Mortensen NJ Mechanism of action of botulinum toxin on the internal anal sphincter. *Br. J. Surg.* 2004;91:224-228.
[35] Kiyak G, Korukluoğlu B, Kuşdemir A, Sişman IC, Ergül E. Results of Lateral Internal Sphincterotomy with Open Technique for Chronic Anal Fissure: Evaluation of Complications, Symptom Relief, and Incontinence with Long-Term Follow-Up. *Dig. Dis. Sci.* 2009 Jan 1. (Epub ahead of print).
[36] Littlejohn DR, Newstead GL. Tailored lateral sphincterotomy for anal fissure. *Dis. Colon Rectum* 1997;40:1439-42.
[37] Fruehauf H, Fried M, Wegmueller B, Bauerfeind P, Thumshirn M. Efficacy and Safety of Botulinum Toxin A Injection Compared with Topical Nitroglycerin Ointment for the treatment of Chronic Anal Fissure: A Prospective Randomized Study. *Am. J. Gastroenterol.* 2006 Sep;101(9):2107-12.
[38] Floyd DN., Kondylis L., Kondylis PD, Reilly JC. Chronic anal fissure: 1994 and a decade later- are we doing better? *Am. J. Surg.* 2006 (191); 344-8
[39] Utzig MJ, Kroesen AJ, Buhr HJ. Concepts in pathogenesis and treatment of chronic anal fissure. A review of the literature. *Am. J. Gastroenterol.* 2003;98:968-74.
[40] Lorder PB, Kamm MA, Nicholls RJ, Philips RK. Reversible chemical sphincterotomy by local application of glyceryl trinitrate. *Br. J. Surg.* 1994;81:1386-9.
[41] Scholefield JH, Bock JU,Marla B, et al. A dose finding study with 0.1 percent,0.2 percent, and 0.4 percent glyceryl trinitrate ointment in patients with chronic anal fissures. *Gut.* 2003;52:264-9.
[42] Zuberi BF, Rajput MR,Abro H, et al. A randomized trial of glyceryl trinitrate ointment and nitroglycerin patch in healing of anal fissures. *Int. J. Colorectal. Dis.* 2000 ;15 :243-5.

[43] Altomare DF, Rinaldi M, Milito G, et al. Glyceryl trinitrate for chronic anal fissure-Healing or headache? Results of a multicenter, randomized, placebo-controlled, double-blind trial. *Dis. Colon Rectum* 2000;43:174-9.
[44] De Naedi P, Ortolano E,Radaelli G, Staudacher C. Comparison of glycerine trinitrate and botulinum Toxin-A for the treatment of chronic anal fissure: Long-term results. Dis. Colon Rectum. 2006 Apr ;49(4) : 427-32.
[45] Schiano di Visconte M, Di Bella R, Munegato G. Randomized, Prospective trial comparino 0.25 percent glycerin trinitrate ointment and anal cryothermal dialtors only with 0.25 percent glycerin trinitrate ointment and only with anal cryothermal dilators in the treatment of chronic anal fissure: a two-year follow-up. *Dis. Colon Rectum* 2006;49:1822-1830.
[46] Brisinda G, Maria G, Bentivoglio AR, Cassetta E, Gui D, Albanese A. A Comparison of injections of botulinum toxin and topical nitroglycerin ointment for the treatment of chronic anal fissure. *N. Engl. J. Med.* 1999;341:65-9.
[47] Witte ME, Klaase JM. Botulinum toxin A injection in ISDN ointment-resistant chronic anal fissures. *Dig. Surg.* 2007;24(3):197-201. Epub 2007 May 15.
[48] Jost WH. One hundred cases of anal fissure treated with botulin toxin: early and long-term results. *Dis. Colon Rectum*. 1997 Sep;40(9):1029-32.
[49] Brisinda G, Maria G, Sganga G, Bentivoglio AR, Albanese A, Castagneto M. Effectiveness of higher doses of botulinum toxin to induce healing in patients with chronic anal fissures. *Surgery*. 2002 Feb;131(2):179-84.
[50] Baraza W, Boereboom C, Shorthouse A, Brown S. The long-term efficacy of fissurectomy and botulinum toxin injection for chronic anal fissure in females. *Dis. Colon Rectum*. 2008 Feb;51(2):239-43. Epub 2008 Jan 4.
[51] Radwan MM, Ramdan K, Abu-Azab I, Abu-Zidan FM. Botulinum toxin treatment for anal fissure. *Afr. Health Sci.* 2007 Mar;7(1):14-7.
[52] Arthur JD, Makin CA, El-Sayed TY, Walsh CJ. A pilot comparative study of fissurectomy/diltiazem and fissurectomy/botulinum toxin the treatment of chronic anal fissure. *Tech. Coloproctol*. 2008 Dec;12(4):331-6; discussion 336.
[53] Smith M, Frizelle F. Long-term faecal incontinence following the use of botulinum toxin. *Colorectal Dis*. 2004 Nov;6(6):526-7
[54] Jost WH, Schrank B. Repeat botulin toxin injections in anal fissure: in patients with relapse and after insufficient effect of first treatment. *Dig. Dis. Sci.* 1999 Aug;44(8):1588-9.
[55] Jones OM, Ramalingam T, Merrie A, Cunningham C, George BD, Mortensen NJ, Lindsey I. Randomized clinical trial of botulinum toxin plus

glyceryl trinitrate vs. botulinum toxin alone for medically resistant chronic anal fissure: overall poor healing rates. *Dis. Colon Rectum.* 2006 Oct;49(10):1574-80.

[56] Maria G, Brisinda G, Bentivoglio AR, Cassetta E, Gui D, Albanese A. Influence of botulinum toxin site of injections on healing rate in patients with chronic anal fissure. *Am. J. Surg.* 2000 Jan;179(1):46-50.

[57] Fernandez LF, Conde FR, Rios RA, Garcia Iglesias J, Cainzos FM, Potel LJ. Botulinum toxin for the treatment oh anal fissure. *Dig. Surg.*1999; 16:515-8.

[58] Minguez M, Herreros B, Espi A, Garcia-Granero E, Sanchiz V, Mora F, Lledo S, Benages A. Long-term follow-up (42 months) of chronic anal fissure after healing with botulinum toxin. *Gastroenterology.* 2002;123:112-7.

[59] Arroyo A, Perez F, Serrano P, Candela F, Lacueva J, Calpena R. Surgical versus chemical (botulinum toxin) sphincterotomy for chronic anal fissure: long-term results of a prospective randomized clinical and manometric study. *Am. J. Surg.* 2005;189:429-34.

[60] Mentes BB, Irkorucu O, Akin M, Leventoglu S, Tatlicioglu E. Comparison of botulinum toxin injection and lateral internal sphincterotomy for the treatment of chronic anal fissure. *Dis. Colon Rectum.* 2003;46:232-7.

[61] Scholz T, Hetzer FH, Dindo D, Demartines N, Clavien PA, Hahnloser D. Long-term follow-up after combined fissurectomy and Botox injection for chronic anal fissures. *Int. J. Colorectal Dis.* 2007 Jan 30.

INDEX

A

access, 22
accommodation, 14
acetylcholine, 48, 49
achalasia, 83, 88
acid, 32
action potential, 15
adaptability, 12
adaptation, 16
adolescents, 93
adrenoceptors, 39
adults, 19, 35, 92, 106
advancement, 57, 66, 76, 82, 83, 96, 101
adverse effects, 35, 108
aetiology, 55
age, 5, 18, 22, 81, 93, 112
AIDS, 91, 92, 95, 96, 97, 98, 103
alcohols, 32
algorithm, 93
allergic reaction, 83
aminoglycosides, 83
amplitude, 32
anal fissures, vii, 30, 34, 35, 36, 37, 39, 42, 43, 44, 45, 55, 56, 59, 60, 61, 63, 64, 66, 71, 89, 91, 93, 95, 96, 98, 100, 102, 111, 118, 119, 120, 121, 122
analgesic, 108
anaphylaxis, 55, 60

anastomosis, 15
anatomy, 4, 10, 23, 24, 25, 66, 72
angiotensin II, 45
angulation, 63
anorectal abscess, 21
anoscopy, 81, 82
ANS, 85
antibiotic, 71
anus, 7, 9, 22, 23, 63, 66, 79, 82, 96, 103, 117
aorta, 8
apex, 2, 3, 6, 66, 108, 117
appointments, 108
arginine, 29, 38, 39, 41, 45
arteries, 8, 9, 10
arterioles, 111
artery, 8, 9, 119
assessment, 78, 81, 87, 93, 101
asymmetry, 19, 20, 27
asymptomatic, 52, 55, 78
atrophy, 82
authorities, 94
autonomic nervous system, 4, 88
awareness, 96
axon terminals, 53

B

bacillus, 47
back pain, 55

base, 1, 56, 64, 65, 95, 107, 108, 116
baths, vii, 30, 108, 113
behavioral change, 81
beneficial effect, 111
benefits, 107, 108
benign, 25, 96, 97
bias, 70
biopsy, 22, 57, 71
biosynthesis, 45
bleeding, vii, 21, 22, 75, 82, 107
blood, vii, 21, 25, 29, 30, 31, 34, 41, 45, 48, 82, 83, 85, 98, 111, 113, 114, 119
blood flow, vii, 29, 30, 31, 34, 41, 45, 98, 111, 113, 114, 119
blood supply, 119
blood vessels, 30
bone, 7
botulism, 48
bowel, 22, 30, 31, 66, 70, 82, 92, 93, 94, 102, 107, 108
breast feeding, 83
breathing, 85

C

calcium, 29, 37, 38, 41, 53, 94, 105, 107, 111, 113
calcium channel blocker, 29, 37, 41, 53, 94, 105, 107, 113
cancer, 22, 107
candidates, 100
capillary, 8
carcinoma, 92, 103
cataract, 69
catheter, 19
cerebral cortex, 14
channel blocker, 29, 37, 41, 53, 94, 105, 107, 113
chemical, vii, 30, 39, 41, 59, 70, 85, 88, 106, 115, 120, 122
Chicago, ix, 63
children, 93
clinical application, 47, 48, 60
clinical disorders, 88
clinical examination, 78

clinical trials, 81, 105, 116
closure, 118
coccyx, 2, 3, 6, 7
colic, 9, 12
colon, 4, 9, 22, 23, 25, 102, 103
colorectal surgeon, 101
colostomy, 12
commercial, 49
commissure, 111
communication, 10
community, 95
complement, 17
complexity, 12
compliance, 12, 13, 18, 35, 36, 38, 47, 53, 96, 113, 114, 115
complications, vii, 55, 70, 75, 94, 97, 101, 102, 107, 108, 111, 112, 116
composition, 23, 30, 58
compression, 111
confinement, 66
connective tissue, 8
consensus, 91, 96, 115
constipation, 17, 41, 82, 99, 100, 111
contracture, 64, 66, 72
control group, 50
controlled trials, 59, 83, 94
controversial, 40, 54, 57
correlation, 22, 97
cortex, 14
cost, 113
coughing, 14
critical value, 16
criticism, 6
cure, 57, 71
cyanotic, 93
cytokines, 98

D

defecation, 12, 14, 16, 17, 18, 20, 21, 24, 25, 26, 66, 96, 100
defects, 19, 20, 24, 64, 67, 71, 75, 80, 81, 83, 112
deficiencies, 19
degradation, 40

destruction, 15, 96, 112
detectable, 83, 85
detection, 17
diaphragm, 3, 7, 24
diarrhea, 94
diet, vii, 30, 82, 100, 108
diffusion, 83
dilation, 64, 65, 71, 72, 110
disability, 67
discomfort, 98, 110, 114
discontinuity, 21
discrimination, 16
disease activity, 102
diseases, 19, 21, 22, 30, 48, 58, 85, 92
disorder, 63, 66
distribution, 1, 15, 119
dogs, 4
donors, 29, 32, 41
dosage, 38, 57, 113, 115
dosing, 43
double-blind trial, 42, 121
drainage, 10, 76
drugs, 30
duodenum, 31
durability, 17

E

ecchymosis, 111
ectropion, 82
education, 96
election, 34
electromyography (EMG), 15, 17, 20, 83
endocrine, 3
enemas, 82
environmental factors, 16
enzyme, 40
epithelium, 2, 3, 12
equipment, 18
esophageal achalasia, 83
esophagus, 12
ESR, 72
etiology, 100
evacuation, 21, 82, 99
evidence, 57, 94, 106, 114, 116

evolution, 102
examinations, 22
excision, 63, 65, 66, 82, 108
exocytosis, 48
exposure, 21, 82
expulsion, 12
extraction, 17
extraocular muscles, 57

F

faecal incontinence, 60, 76, 80, 86, 87, 100, 115, 121
fascia, 5, 23
fat, 5
fear, 71, 106
fears, 97
feces, 76, 83, 115
feelings, 13
fiber, vii, 30, 93, 100, 113
fibers, 3, 4, 5, 7, 8, 11, 12, 13, 15, 30, 64, 65, 78, 82, 111
fibrosis, 56, 57, 107, 115, 116
fistulas, 71, 76, 102
fluid, 78
force, 12, 18
formation, 13, 64
foundations, 25
friction, 16
fusion, 48

G

gangrene, 55, 60
gastric mucosa, 3
gastrointestinal tract, 31
gel, 38, 39, 44, 45, 107
gender differences, 19
general anaesthesia, 54
general practitioner, vii
geometry, 19
glycerin, 121
grading, 87
growth, 53

guidelines, 94

H

hair, 3
headache, 29, 35, 38, 41, 42, 110, 113, 114, 121
health, 43
heart block, 83, 88
heart disease, 39
heart rate, 85
hematoma, 83
hemorrhage, 21, 112
hemorrhoids, 21, 22, 24, 72, 92, 98, 102, 103
hemostasis, 67
heterogeneity, 34
heterosexuals, 95
high risk patients, 106
histology, 60
history, 16, 20, 22, 30, 34, 56, 79, 92, 98, 101, 107
HIV, 91, 92, 95, 96, 97, 98, 103
HIV/AIDS, 91, 92, 95, 98
homosexuals, 103
hospitalization, 66
human, 15, 25, 27, 31, 45, 58, 102, 103
human immunodeficiency virus, 102, 103
human subjects, 27
hypertension, 39
hypotension, 35, 83
hypothesis, 15, 98

I

ICC, 4
identification, 19, 101
idiopathic, 59, 87, 88, 92, 96, 118
immunodeficiency, 95, 102, 103
improvements, 34
impulses, 14
in vitro, 49, 58
in vivo, 49, 58

incidence, 9, 29, 35, 37, 52, 57, 68, 69, 70, 75, 76, 78, 81, 82, 86, 91, 92, 95, 98, 99, 100, 110, 112, 113, 119
individuals, 19, 96
induration, 78, 93
infection, 64, 71, 95, 96, 102, 103, 107
inflammation, 93, 95
inflammatory bowel disease, 22, 30, 93, 94, 107
ingestion, 48
inguinal, 10
inhibition, 16, 40
inhibitor, 40
injections, 35, 43, 54, 55, 58, 59, 60, 85, 89, 106, 115, 121, 122
injuries, 21, 65, 101
insertion, 7
integrity, 20, 21
intercourse, 96
interference, 48, 101
intervention, 71, 91, 92, 95, 96, 97
intestine, 9, 31
intrinsic precursor, 38
intussusception, 20, 56, 61
ionizing radiation, 20
Ireland, 84
iron, 100
ischaemic heart disease, 39
ischemia, 9, 64
ischium, 7
islands, 3
issues, 47, 53, 113, 115
Italy, ix, x, 1, 29, 75, 91, 105, 107, 108

K

kill, 49

L

laceration, 100
L-arginine, 29, 38, 39, 41, 45
laxatives, vii, 30, 50, 82
lead, 33, 66

leakage, 17, 78
lesions, 20, 91, 93, 97, 98, 99, 100, 103
levator, 3, 4, 5, 6, 7, 11, 12, 15, 25
ligament, 3, 6, 7, 11, 23
light, 37, 48
local anesthesia, 79, 115, 118
localization, 20, 98
lumen, 1
lymph, 10
lymph node, 10
lymphocytes, 98

M

magnetic resonance imaging (MRI), 5, 17, 20, 82
majority, 64, 69, 91, 92, 98
malignancy, 57
man, 24, 25, 26, 55, 58, 60
management, vii, 42, 61, 63, 64, 72, 81, 82, 92, 94, 95, 101, 102, 103, 120
matter, 12, 16, 114
measurement, 13, 17, 79, 85
measurements, 18, 79
median, 8, 80, 98, 99
medical, vii, 22, 29, 35, 38, 39, 41, 71, 75, 78, 81, 86, 92, 94, 95, 97, 101, 105, 106, 107, 108, 109, 110, 111, 113, 116, 117
medical history, 22
medication, 71
menopause, 52
mesenteric vessels, 10
meta-analysis, 50, 52, 59, 76, 105
metabolized, 32
mice, 49
morbidity, 34, 75, 86, 96, 97, 111, 117
morphology, 30, 82
motor neurons, 32
mucosa, 2, 3, 15, 16, 22, 95, 96, 98, 111
multivariate analysis, 42, 61
muscarinic receptor, 15
muscle relaxation, 39, 40, 114
muscles, 4, 6, 7, 8, 9, 12, 14, 15, 17, 21, 25, 26, 57, 83
myasthenia gravis, 83

myasthenic syndrome, 83
myosin, 37

N

narcotic, 108
nerve, 7, 8, 10, 11, 12, 13, 15, 16, 17, 25, 26, 48, 49, 54, 58
nerve fibers, 11
nervous system, 4, 19, 32, 88
neurons, 15, 31, 32
neuropathy, 20
neurotransmitter, 31, 111
nitrates, 31, 32, 35, 36, 38, 42, 43, 58, 84, 89, 94, 107
nitric oxide, 29, 31, 32, 38, 41, 52, 58, 113
nodes, 10, 48
nucleoside analogs, 96
nucleotides, 40

O

obstruction, 10
oesophageal, 31
operations, 25, 95, 97
organ, 49, 82
organs, 6, 11
outpatients, 118

P

pain, vii, 15, 21, 22, 29, 34, 38, 41, 55, 66, 69, 75, 81, 82, 91, 93, 96, 107, 113, 114
paralysis, 48, 115
paresthesias, 71
pathogenesis, 85, 86, 116, 119, 120
pathology, 92, 93, 97, 102
pathophysiological, 48, 82
pathophysiology, 55, 94
pathways, 31
pelvic floor, 1, 10, 12, 14, 15, 16, 20, 21, 24, 25, 26, 58, 100
pelvis, 10
penis, 11

perfusion, 82, 113
perianal abscess, 111
perineum, 3, 6, 22, 99
periosteum, 7
permeability, 32
pharmacokinetics, 32, 42
pharmacological treatment, 106
pharmacology, 26, 49
Philadelphia, 23, 24, 26
physiological mechanisms, 16
physiology, 17, 18, 24, 25, 27, 48, 49, 57, 58
physiopathology, 100
pigs, 49
pilot study, 41, 61
placebo, 33, 34, 35, 38, 42, 45, 50, 105, 113, 116, 121
plexus, 3, 8, 10, 11, 12, 13, 16, 19, 31
poison, 60
polypeptides, 48
population, vii, 15, 39, 64, 93, 94, 96, 97
postural hypotension, 83
pregnancy, 83, 91, 92, 98, 99, 100, 103
preparation, 49, 84, 107, 108
preservation, 24
pressure gradient, 13, 19
probe, 17, 20
proctitis, 94
proctoscopy, 22, 81, 82
prognosis, 96
prolapse, 20, 56, 57
prolapsed, 27, 82
prophylaxis, 96
protease inhibitors, 96
pruritus, vii, 75, 82, 110, 113, 114
pruritus ani, 110, 114
pubis, 6
puerperium, 98, 100

Q

quality of life, 76, 81
quantification, 24
questionnaire, 70

R

radiation, 20, 21, 82, 112
reactions, 83
receptors, 14, 15, 16, 40
recognition, 31
recovery, 48, 113
rectal prolapse, 20, 27
rectocele, 20
rectum, 1, 2, 3, 4, 5, 6, 8, 9, 10, 11, 12, 13, 14, 15, 16, 18, 22, 23, 25, 26, 58, 93, 103, 119
recurrence, 30, 38, 39, 42, 64, 66, 68, 70, 71, 76, 78, 81, 85, 106, 110, 111, 113, 114, 115, 116, 117
reflexes, 14, 16, 83
relapses, 53, 113
relaxation, 13, 14, 15, 16, 18, 31, 32, 39, 40, 49, 56, 58, 100, 111, 113, 114
relief, vii, 30, 38, 39, 67, 81, 113
renin, 40, 45
repair, 83
reparation, 84, 108
resection, 61
resistance, 16, 18, 92, 102
resolution, 57
respiratory failure, 48
response, 14, 15, 18, 26, 49, 56, 61, 70, 81, 85, 100, 101, 106, 112
risk, vii, 20, 22, 29, 30, 34, 35, 40, 71, 80, 81, 85, 91, 94, 99, 100, 105, 106, 112, 113, 116, 117
risk factors, 22, 30, 34
risks, 52, 95, 100, 101, 108
roots, 10, 11, 15

S

sacrum, 3, 6, 7
safety, 30, 40, 47, 55, 57, 85, 113, 116
scar tissue, 56
seed, 100
sensation, 12, 18, 26
sensitivity, 12, 19, 82

serum, 22
sexually transmitted diseases, 22
shame, 78
shape, 63
showing, 9, 13, 39, 67
side effects, 29, 31, 35, 36, 38, 39, 41, 44, 47, 52, 57, 70, 83, 107, 110, 113, 115, 116
signals, 16
signs, 39, 78
single chain, 48
sitz baths, vii, 30, 108
skin, 2, 3, 5, 6, 32, 63, 64, 65, 66, 72, 82, 83, 91, 93, 97, 98, 107, 116
small intestine, 9, 31
smooth muscle, 4, 5, 8, 13, 31, 32, 37, 39, 40, 45, 48, 58, 111
smooth muscle cells, 32
softener, 108
solution, 108
South Asia, 39
spastic, 21, 64
specific knowledge, 91
specifications, 34
spinal cord, 10, 15
spine, 2, 7
sprouting, 48
state, 14, 15, 32, 85, 94
states, 12, 16, 96
stenosis, 82, 85
steroids, 94
stimulus, 14
stomach, 31
strabismus, 48, 57
structural changes, 66
structure, 7, 12, 25, 58
submucosa, 1, 3, 8, 9, 12
substrate, 15
success rate, 114
supplementation, 93, 100
surface area, 32
surface layer, 6
surgical intervention, 71, 91, 96, 97
surgical technique, 12, 76, 79
suture, 67
symmetry, 19

sympathetic fibers, 11
sympathetic nerve fibers, 11
symptoms, 21, 22, 29, 34, 52, 55, 57, 70, 75, 78, 87, 88, 92, 107, 108
syndrome, 21, 61, 83
syphilis, 92

T

T cell, 98
tabes dorsalis, 15
target, 30
techniques, 12, 16, 63, 76, 86, 112
telephone, 78
tendon, 5
tension, 15, 16
terminals, 53, 115
test scores, 85
testing, 17, 18, 81
tetanus, 58
textbook, 88
therapy, 22, 29, 30, 36, 41, 42, 44, 47, 52, 54, 59, 71, 86, 88, 93, 94, 95, 97, 101, 106, 107, 110, 113, 116, 117, 118
thrombosis, 83
tissue, 5, 8, 11, 56, 64, 82, 108, 115, 116
tonic, 14, 15, 49
transection, 15
transmission, 83, 88
trauma, 66, 95, 96, 111, 112
traumatic events, 98, 99
trial, 33, 34, 36, 37, 38, 39, 42, 43, 44, 45, 50, 52, 53, 58, 60, 64, 65, 70, 72, 87, 88, 93, 103, 106, 117, 118, 120, 121
tuberculosis, 92
tumors, 21

U

ulcer, 22, 40, 61, 76, 98, 112
ultrasonography, 4, 20, 21, 79, 80, 82, 87
ultrasound, 17, 20, 56, 57, 72, 81, 112
United, x, 34, 66, 95
United Kingdom (UK), x, 38, 44, 54, 84

United States (USA), 34, 63, 66, 84, 95
urethra, 3
urinary bladder, 58
urinary retention, 111, 112
urine, 83

V

variations, 13, 14, 18, 76
vascularization, 8, 9
vector, 19, 20
vein, 10
vessels, 8, 10, 30
Viagra, 45
virus infection, 102
viscoelastic properties, 25

W

waste, 14
water, vii, 30, 100, 107
weakness, 82, 83
withdrawal, 35, 39
workers, 38, 75, 76, 85
wound healing, 66, 67, 82, 94, 96, 97, 98, 103

Y

young adults, 92
young women, 55